The International Library of Psychology

PERSONALITY

Founded by C. K. Ogden

The International Library of Psychology

INDIVIDUAL DIFFERENCES
In 21 Volumes

I	The Practice and Theory of Individual Psychology	*Adler*
II	The Neurotic Constitution	*Adler*
III	Duality	*Bradley*
IV	Problems of Personality	*Campbell et al*
V	An Introduction to Individual Psychology	*Dreikurs*
VI	The Psychology of Alfred Adler and the Development of the Child	*Ganz*
VII	Personality	*Gordon*
VIII	The Art of Interrogation	*Hamilton*
IX	Appraising Personality	*Harrower*
X	Physique and Character	*Kretschmer*
XI	The Psychology of Men of Genius	*Kretschmer*
XII	Handreading	*Laffan*
XIII	On Shame and the Search for Identity	*Lynd*
XIV	A B C of Adler's Psychology	*Mairet*
XV	Alfred Adler: Problems of Neurosis	*Mairet*
XVI	Principles of Experimental Psychology	*Piéron*
XVII	The Psychology of Character	*Roback*
XVIII	The Hands of Children	*Spier*
XIX	The Nature of Intelligence	*Thurstone*
XX	Alfred Adler: The Pattern of Life	*Wolfe*
XXI	The Psychology of Intelligence and Will	*Wyatt*

PERSONALITY

R G GORDON

Routledge
Taylor & Francis Group
LONDON AND NEW YORK

First published in 1926 by
Kegan Paul, Trench, Trubner & Co., Ltd.

Published in 2001 by
Routledge
2 Park Square, Milton Park, Abingdon, Oxfordshire OX14 4RN
711 Third Avenue, New York, NY 10017

First issued in paperback 2014

Routledge is an imprint of the Taylor and Francis Group, an informa business

British Library Cataloguing in Publication Data
A CIP catalogue record for this book
is available from the British Library

Personality
ISBN 978-0415-21057-7
Individual Differences: 21 Volumes
ISBN 0415-21130-1
The International Library of Psychology: 204 Volumes
ISBN 0415-19132-7

ISBN 978-1-138-87538-8 (pbk)
ISBN 978-0-415-21057-7 (hbk)

CONTENTS

PREFACE

THE publication of this book seems to need some explanation. Why should a practising physician write on personality? Should not this task be undertaken by an erudite psychologist, who is *au fait* with all the intricacies of mental science. The answer may be, that Personality is essentially a practical entity and not a theoretical composition. Moreover, the physician, especially if he practise amongst those who are instable in body and mind, is constantly brought up against all sorts and conditions of personalities. He must study these personalities with care, he must analyse, to find out what are the symptoms of ill-health, yet he must never lose sight of the total synthesis. To treat individual symptoms is futile, to treat the patient as a whole, in all his relations, individual and social, is essential. Thus a conception of personality is gained, which is rather different from that of the professional psychologist. It is in the hope that this conception, however inadequately expressed, may be of some interest and use, that this task has been undertaken. Only in a few cases have quotations from authorities been inserted verbatim, but many ideas and opinions have been borrowed from the writings of others. So far as possible, these have been acknowledged, by the references to their works at the end of the book. These references may also enable those, who find certain passages obscure, to pursue the subject further, as the reader's general acquaintance with the more modern neurological and psychological literature has been assumed, in order to keep the book with a reasonable compass.

But for the influence of certain men who taught me Neurology and Psychology, this task would have been quite impossible, and I would like to express my indebtedness, especially to Sir Byrom Bramwell, to Professors Lloyd Morgan and T. H. Pear, and to Drs A. F. Hurst, the late R. G. Rows, and Bernard Hart. Also the suggestions and criticisms of Drs R. W. Lang Todd, L. G. Irvine, and other friends have been of the greatest value.

Finally, I am indebted to the painstaking care and patience of Miss Bickerstaff, for the preparation of the manuscript and the correction of proofs.

PERSONALITY

CHAPTER I

INTRODUCTION

MANY psychologists have endeavoured to present an adequate explanation of Personality, but it still remains a somewhat vague conception, such as is beloved by the journalist, since he may twist it to fit any meaning he chooses. To define the term is a matter of difficulty, for Personality is one of those concepts which all of us take for granted as having a concise meaning, until we try to express that meaning in words. One reason of this difficulty is that most definitions are given in terms of the component parts of the whole, whereas Personality can only have a meaning if thought of in terms of a synthesis. The first and most general impulse of mankind when he wants to understand is to take the watch to pieces, to see how the wheels go round. It is only later and in certain cases that there is any enthusiasm to put it together again and understand its construction. Apart from this, however, few people, except those who have given special study to the subject, are at all clear as to what they wish to define when they talk of Personality. The difference between such terms as the ego, the character, and the personality, is not realized, and they are apt to become interchangeable. Before proceeding further it would be well to distinguish between these terms.

The term *ego* is not a strictly scientific expression, and it is used somewhat loosely even in scientific works. However it is constantly met with in psychological literature, and a definition must be attempted. It is used to describe the purely personal attributes of any individual, which mark him off from other objects in his environment and other selves in the community. In Chapter VII reference is made to McDougall's work [1] and to the concept of the

A

self-regarding sentiment.* The development of this sentiment and the attendant functions of self-consciousness and reflective thought are the essential factors in the establishment of the ego, as a conscious entity in the life of the individual. By the organization of this sentiment the subject is contrasted and marked off from his objective environment, and at the same time is related to his surroundings. The contrast is appreciated, between what I am and what you are, between what I feel and what you feel, and the term ego also has reference to the aims and tendencies of the individual in relation to his environment. These aims have an intimately personal purpose. Thus we may talk of ego impulses and ego ideals when we mean activities and goals which shall redound to the greater glorification and intensity of pleasure of the individual himself, or which may bring about that position in respect to his environment which he himself wishes to occupy, quite apart from his altruistic or social commitments.

By the term *character* we mean the dominant sentiments and beliefs of an individual at any given time, whereby his attitude to himself and his environment is determined. It is abundantly clear that these dominant sentiments and beliefs by no means constitute the whole personality and that character may change according to the environment, whether temporal or spatial, in which the individual finds himself. A sudden access of wealth, the loss of a loved one, or the mere passage of years, may totally change the character of the man. Indeed, he may present two characters coincidently, for his character at home may be that of a model husband and father, while abroad he may be quite the reverse. Nor need this be a wholly hypocritical state of affairs, for in the environment of home his dominant sentiment may be love of family for the time being, while abroad other sentiments may take the lead. Inasmuch as character is the source of behaviour which can be observed by others, it is comparatively easy to infer. Hence we may rightly talk of giving a person a character. The accuracy of such a character will depend on whether our observation is

* A sentiment is an organization of emotional dispositions in relation to an object and will be discussed in Chapter VII. Sentiments may be exemplified by love for a person, hate of a person, keenness on golf, etc. The self-regarding sentiment has the self for the object and involves the function of self-consciousness.

reliable, and whether we have had a reasonable opportunity of watching the person's behaviour under a variety of circumstances and over a long period of time. Even so, we cannot guarantee that the character we give will be accurate, unless the person is likely to be in an environment similar to that in which we have watched him.

Personality, on the other hand, is a much more complex matter, and includes the ego and the character. It involves all the heredity of the individual; that is, all the bodily and mental dispositions, both actual and potential, with which he is equipped at birth. The factor of heredity is at present somewhat out of the picture in psychology. The reason for this is that the interest in the study of the subject, which was so prominent at the end of last century, revealed so many problems and difficulties that a quiescent period of further experiment was required to prove or disprove the theories advanced. Except in so far as any characteristic can be definitely recognized as a Mendelian dominant, it is hard to predict its transmissibility. The recognition of such dominants is hard enough in bodily structure, but in mental function it is almost impossible to elucidate them. Moreover, in the generality of mankind the stock is so mixed that in a few generations even the most transmissible characters are soon swamped, and it is difficult to trace any continuity of succession with any scientific exactitude except in certain royal or aristocratic families such as the Hapsburgs, Stuarts and others, in whom a special bodily characteristic can be recognized through several generations. Yet, although transmissibility of bodily and mental character cannot be predicted or even recognized with certainty, every individual does owe a great deal to his forebears. In the first place, it will be generally conceded that race is of great importance. However similar the environment, the personalities of the Aryan, the Mongol and the Negro can never be the same. Secondly, such factors as stature, bodily strength and resistance to disease, both generally and particularly, are unquestionably transmissible and make all the difference to the individual in his contact with his environment. Thirdly, there are factors in character, the impulses that dominate the behaviour of the personality, which are transmitted from father to son. Although such an idea as that contained in Mr. Buchan's *Path of the King*[1] may not be scientific, undoubtedly it contains a great deal of truth. In this book "he sees the younger sons carry the royal blood far down among the people, down even into the kennels of the outcast. . . . Some rags of greatness always cling to it, the dumb faith that, sometime and somehow, that blood drawn from kings it never knew will be royal again. Though nature is wasteful of material things there is no waste of spirit." In Chapter VI attention will be drawn to the dispositions which constitute the equipment, with which each individual starts out in life, but though these may be qualitatively common to all humanity, they are not so quantitatively, and their variations are determined by heredity. Abnormalities in their relative proportion are of great importance in determining behaviour, and as will be seen later, character may be so constituted as a result of such abnormalities that the adjustment to the environment is impossible.

To the inherited factors in personality must be added all the modifications which have been impressed upon the individual from his environment. Some of these are brought about before birth, but the full nature and extent of prenatal influences are still obscure. The developing embryo is peculiarly well protected from external influence, except through the circulating blood of the mother. Legend and popular belief hold it possible that the mental processes of the mother may influence the child, apart from the hereditary transmission of the dispositions; and that various mal-formations, birth marks and so forth, are to be accounted for by her perceptions and emotions during pregnancy. The materialistic science of the 19th century denied the possibility of this, and attributed all cases cited in support of such a theory, to coincidence. In the light of more modern research on the effect of emotional states on the activity of the endocrine glands, and through them on the composition of the blood, it behoves us to be less dogmatic and accept any such theories as being at present unproven. For it may be that the subtle changes induced by these reactions in the mother's blood may have more effect on the malleable tissues of the fœtus than could be induced in the more stable tissues of the adult. Be that as it may, there can be no doubt that more crude and permanent defects or excesses of these secretions in the mother do affect the child, while the transmission of various infections from mother to child is of everyday occurrence. Certain recent work tends to show that the most important period for the transmission of modifications is during the first six weeks of fœtal life. At this period the function of the adrenal glands has not commenced in the embryo, and in consequence resistance to extraneous chemical substances is at a minimum; for the products of these glands seem to exercise a definite protective influence against foreign toxins. After the sixth week modifications are much less frequent and extraneous agencies much less potent. Unfortunately, it is just in the first six weeks that it is most difficult to protect the embryo from harm since the mother often does not know that she is pregnant and therefore does not take the precautions she might otherwise exercise. Nor is it easy in these early stages to establish exactly what changes do occur and what poisons or endocrine modifications are significant. In the present state of our knowledge therefore we must keep an open mind as to the effects of maternal perceptions and emotions in the early stages of pregnancy, but we are probably right in adopting a sceptical attitude towards the effects of impressions in the later months.

Relatively to influences after birth however, prenatal modifications of the personality are not important. These other influences continue to act on the individual with greater or less effect all through life. The nature of these will depend on the race and the social position of the individual, on the composition of his family, on his educational menage, on the career he chooses, or which is chosen for him, on marriage, on children, and on the whole gamut of his social relationship. Still, the most striking and lasting modifications will occur in childhood and adolescence. At this time he is malleable both in body and mind. An illness may permanently affect his growth, an alarming experience may permanently modify his attitude towards a whole series of his reactions. If he is the object of too persistent love, indifference, or cruelty, his emotional attitudes may be so warped that he can never free himself from these early influences. The older he grows, the more violent must the accidents of fortune be if they are to make a lasting impression, and as life progresses and habits of thought and action become more fixed, the more difficult is it to influence the personality for good or ill. Personality also involves all the subtle relationships between the individual and the environment in so far as his actions modify the latter. That is to say, we are concerned, not only with the incoming impressions, but also with the outgoing impulses of the individual, which depend not only on the organization of the personality, but also on the situation in the environment which he requires to meet. We see, therefore, that so far as this study is concerned, a much more comprehensive purview is required than when the ego alone is dealt with. Indeed, we may say that to define a man's personality adequately, we must describe his parentage and race, his bodily structure, his intellectual attainments, his emotional reactions, his practical achievement, and all the slings and arrows of outrageous fortune that have fallen upon him from birth to death. We must know the answer to the riddles whence man came, what he is and whither he is going. In other words we should require an encyclopædia of all the sciences and philosophies to serve our ends completely. Since it is impossible to accomplish such a task in full, no more than a brief sketch can be attempted, but we may describe in outline how his bodily structure is correlated with his mental reactions and how each relates to the environment. From these is established that unity which we recognize as personality. If this sketch, inadequate though it may be, serves to clarify to some extent the hazy ideas on the subject which are current, something will have been achieved.

What man is and how man became what he is were questions so vital, once self-consciousness was evolved, that they were bound to exercise the human mind from the earliest times. Long before the era of history, primitive man in his folk-lore and fairy tales attempted to explain his origin and existence. As Laing[3] has pointed out, there were three possible explanations of how man took his place in the world; that he was formed from inanimate objects, that he was descended from animals, or that he was created by supernatural agencies. The attribution of magical qualities to stones and trees made it feasible to the primitive mind that these sticks and stones might be changed into men and women, and conversely human beings might be changed to stones. The myth of Deucalion and Pyrrha illustrates this. The story is the Greek version of the Biblical flood. The aged Deucalion and Pyrrha built themselves a stout ship, whereby they survived the deluge. But when the water had subsided they found themselves stranded in a gorge at the mouth of a cave which was afterwards known as Delphi. In spite of their relief at their salvation they grieved that they, old and childless, were the sole survivors of man on earth. However, in the midst of their despair, Themis appeared in a dream and bade them have courage. "If you would see human faces about you once more, O Deucalion and Pyrrha, then take and cast behind you the bones of your Great Mother." On waking, they were perplexed at first as to what this oracle meant, but soon they understood that by bones of the Great Mother were meant the rocks of earth. So each gathered a lap-ful of stones and cast them behind them. Each stone that Deucalion threw changed into a man and each of Pyrrha's into a woman and so the whole earth was repeopled. Somewhat similar was the story of Cadmus. Expelled from his father's house to find his lost sister Europa, who had been carried off by Zeus, in the guise of a bull, he and his two slaves came to a cave where dwelt a dragon. Cadmus sent the slaves to search the cave, but they never returned, for they were slain by the dragon. However, Cadmus himself overcame and killed the beast, but finding himself alone, despaired of obeying the oracle who had commanded him to build a city. Minerva thereupon appeared and told him to plough up the place and sow the dragon's teeth. From each there quickly grew a warrior in full armour. These turned on each other and fought desperately, till all were slain but five, who, deeming it wiser to desist, made friends with Cadmus and helped him to build the city, which was afterwards known to fame as Thebes. The reverse transformation of men and women into stones, is illustrated by the myth of Daphne, changed into a tree—the laurel of Apollo—by her father, the river-god, to protect her from the amorous pursuit of her lover; by the story of Lot's wife turned to a pillar of salt for looking back at the burning cities, and by the Cornish maidens who became a circle of stones in punishment for dancing on the Sabbath.

The origin of man from animals is found in the totem beliefs so common among primitive man. "It is a step in advance of the pure fetish worship of stocks and stones, to conceive of animals, as having thought and language, and being in fact men under a different form. From this it is a short step to endowing them with magical attributes and supernatural powers, adopting them as patrons of tribes and families and finally considering them as ancestors."[4] The totem ancestor of the tribe—the fox, the beaver, the bear, the eagle and so on,—distinguishes it from all other clans and is supposed to endow its members with the wisdom, strength, courage or other attributes of the ancestral animal. Marriage with another member of the totem is incestuous, and many taboos have direct reference to relationship with the animal ancestor of the tribe. The transformation of men into animals and animals into men is too common in myth and fairy story to necessitate the quotation of examples; for the frogs and birds and other animals who were really handsome princes or beautiful princesses are familiar to everyone from the nursery.

The belief in the supernatural origin of man may be exemplified by the legend of Bel, who made men out of clay and moulded them with his own blood, and of Jehovah, who fashioned them from the dust and breathed into their nostrils the breath of life.

Primitive man accepted his body as he found it, and strove to explain his mind by reference to the character of his ancestors or creators. In the legends built up on these beliefs we find a firm conviction of the duality of body and mind. To the primitive it seemed obvious common sense that the flesh and the spirit must be two different beings. His stones and rude weapons would not move or work without some agency to make them do so, and why should it be supposed that the body could work unless something or someone is there to work it? We find that he commonly explains the processes of inanimate nature by supposing that they are produced by living beings, working in and behind the phenomena. So a man lives and moves because of the presence of a little man within him, who directs the process. This soul is generally regarded as being fashioned in the likeness of a man. He is supposed to be able to depart from the body, temporarily in sleep and sickness, and permanently in death. The control of bodily structure and function is taken as a matter of course, all deviations from the normal being attributed to the action of the soul. The desire to prevent the departure of the soul from the body was responsible for many of the taboos which surrounded individuals, especially those who were important to the tribe, such as the chiefs and priests. In the belief of many primitives, souls may escape or be lured away from their bodies, by demons or enemies. Certain sorcerers make a living by snaring lost souls, and retailing them at a price to those who had lost them and consequently were sick. It does not seem to matter whether the souls which are purchased are the originals or not, for so long as some soul was returned to the body, recovery from sickness would ensue. Similarly, shadows and reflections were supposed to be the souls of the originals, and damage to the former meant death to the latter. This accounts for the very general fear of the camera met with amongst the lower races of man, since they supposed that the reflections on the plate represent their souls, and that these being taken away they will surely die. The primitive thinks of the personality in terms of this duality. There is his body, of which he is aware, but of whose structure he has only the haziest idea and in which he takes no special interest. This body functions in virtue of its life, which depends on the soul which has a more or less material nature. He cannot conceive of life in abstract terms, but thinks of it as something which can be handled and shut up in a box. He does not think that it need always be actually retained in a body, but it may absent itself therefrom and exert its influence from a distance, provided it remains secure and unharmed; but should it suffer injury, there results sickness and perhaps death of the body.

As we pass from primitive lore to historical philosophy, we find that the dual idea of an essentially separate body and soul still exists. If we take Plato and Aristotle as the culmination of Greek philosophy, we find that their conceptions of personality are essentially dualistic. Plato the idealist, like Socrates, was not interested in nature, so that his conception was necessarily general rather than particular. He insisted on the desirability of a healthy body, which should be trained by music and gymnastics. The soul, however, is divine in origin, but requires contact with the body to find expression. The divine attribute of the universal soul is reason, whose function it is to control the sensuous appetites of the bodily individual soul. Together with these two attributes there exists a third, courage or spirit, by which intermediate link the divine and thc bodily functions are brought into relationship. The ideal personality for Plato, then, is he who by means of divine intellect and reason controls the bodily greeds and lusts. The attitude of Plato towards personality is essentially ethical and not scientific. He is not interested in the nature and constitution of personality in itself, as it concerns us here. Such a conception is more in sympathy with the philosophy of Aristotle, who went to nature for his facts and strove to correlate these in one comprehensive philosophy. He realized the essential unity of the universe and the relation of man to the rest of living beings. He describes nutrition as the function of plants, sensation as that of animals, and locomotion as the function of the higher animals, in an ascending scale. Each of the higher functions involves those below it, and his explanation of the soul is that it is the unification of these various functions of organic life into a single common volitional activity. This soul is inconceivable without the body and the body inconceivable without the soul, while the latter is related to the body as form is to matter. But his dualism emerges in his conception of a fourth power which is quite immaterial and essentially separate from the body. This is the νους, the divine intellect which guides the behaviour of the body and is immortal and eternal. This conception of νους again leads on to the ethical consideration and away from the pure study of personality. We have in the teachings of these two the foundations of idealism and realism in philosophy, but there was no real advance in the study of personality till modern philosophy began with Descartes. The Romans were essentially a non-philosophic people and made no independent contributions to this study, simply adopting the theories of the Greeks and largely depending on Greeks for most of their culture. Nor was an inquiry into the nature of personality encouraged under the influence of mediæval thought or scholastic philosophy, except in so far as the study of the ideal personality of Christ, as an example for all believers, may be held to belong to the subject. Again however, we find that the interest was centred, not on the make up of the personality, but on his ethical value. The philosophic aspect of the subject in more modern times is discussed in outline in the next chapter which deals with the relationship of body and mind, both of which are essential in the synthesis under consideration. With the gradual growth of the sciences of anatomy and physiology during the last three centuries we cannot deal from considerations of space, but their essential contribution to the study of personality is obvious. This is specially the case since the work of Sherrington[5] and others has shown how the nervous system controls and integrates all the functions of the body, and therefore no complete conception of Personality can be arrived at without a knowledge of the structure and function of this system. None the less, it is only recently that the psycho-physical approach has been regarded as desirable or even possible. For the biologist and the physician became more and more materialistic with the advance in knowledge and the apparent simplification of previously abstruse philosophical problems by the work of such men as Darwin and Huxley. On the other hand, philosophers and psychologists have been too prone to stand aloof from the maelstrom of scientific discovery, and, in the seclusion of their studies spin theories from their introspective experiences. Lately, however, the revolt from *a priori* reasoning and the return to the empirical study of facts, has led to an altered relationship between psychology and physiology. On the one hand, the American school of behaviourists and on the other the Austrian and Swiss schools of psycho-analysis have sought to deduce physiological and psychological explanations from observed facts, and have thus been driven towards the necessity of correlating the knowledge of body with that of mind. Moreover, still more recently, a halt has been called in the tendency to seek the explanation of everything by analysis into its component parts, valuable as this method has been. From all sides, in Neurology, Psychology and Philosophy, authorities have begun to study the tendency of a subject as a whole, and to study the complete structure, rather than the elements from which it is composed. In neurology the work of Hughlings Jackson,[6] Sherrington, Head,[7] Rivers,[8] and others has shown how the nervous system works as a whole, organized and integrated together and finally controlled by the cerebral cortex.* They have found that the functions of certain reflex arcs are totally suppressed so far as manifest activity is concerned, yet there can be no doubt that their presence and collaboration are essential to the movement of the whole. Again other reflexes are obviously fused so that the contri-

* *Vide*, Chapter IV.

bution of each to the total function is easily determined. In fact the activity of no part of the nervous system can be considered as having a meaning except in relation to the rest. Thus, when we talk of cortical function, what we really mean is that such and such differences are made in the reactions of the nervous mechanism when the animal develops a cortex. These differences may be studied in man, if the cortex is thrown out of action. But it has no function except in relation to the rest. When the cortex of an animal is removed we have to deal with a new entity, the decerebrate animal, which differs from the complete entity in certain particular respects and is not merely a part of the former. In fact the complete nervous system and the decerebrate nervous system are both unities which react as they do, not in respect of the various nervous arcs into which they can be analysed, but in respect of the relationship of these various arcs to each other and of the constitution of the whole.

In psychology the "Gestalt" theory originated by Wertheimer[9] and developed by several psychologists especially in Germany, prominent among whom are Köhler[10] and Koffka,[11] emphasizes the principle that structural totalities must be the units of mental activity. The chief work of these observers has been done on perception and they have striven to show that perception is not and cannot be merely a bundle of elements of experience, but must possess a unity and structure of its own. For example, suppose we draw a line thus 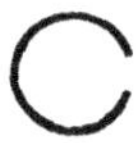 an observer would perceive this as an incomplete circle. That is to say that the circle would be perceived as a whole and then its attribute of incompleteness added. They insist that all perceptions are structural totalities having a definite structure before they can be perceptions. So with all mental processes, they lay stress on the paramount importance of the whole, rather than of the component parts of the organization. This applies to personality with special force, for it is not a mere bundle of sensations, images, wishes, emotions, sentiments, nerve cells. gland activities and so on, but a structural totality, depending not only on these component parts, but on their relatedness to each other and to the whole.

In philosophy, the theories of Alexander[12] and Lloyd

Morgan[13] tend in the same direction. They direct attention to the importance of the new emergent in evolution, as opposed to the constituents into which it may be analysed. The doctrine of emergence, which we shall study in Chapter III does much to overcome the objections which the Animists, such as McDougall,[14] raise to the so-called materialists, viz., that it is absurd to say that a personality is nothing but a collection of tropisms * and conditioned reflexes.† All these enter into the construction of the personality, but the whole nature and life of the latter depend on their organization and relatedness to each other. In virtue of such relatedness, there emerges something new, something distinct, with an individuality of its own. However similar the elements of the personality, their relatedness is certainly different and that is why each individual emerges as a separate unique being. But a personality is not only an emergent from the combination of his bodily and mental attributes, for he cannot exist, except in relation to his environment, in the widest sense of the term. Hence a human being must always be considered in relation to his surroundings if we are to get a comprehensive view. For these reasons the following scheme has been followed in presenting a study of personality. We have to consider the units of which it is made up, and yet always keep in view that these units act as a whole, in virtue of their relatedness to each other and their organization, and that they have no real meaning and little importance as individual entities. Personality might therefore be defined as the emergent synthesis of the bodily and mental attributes of the individual in relation to the environment in the most comprehensive sense.

The relationship of body and mind is the first theme for discussion, with special reference to the theory of emergence which explains how a fresh unity arises. Then the special bodily integration of nervous system and endocrine glands, which forms the purely physical aspect of the study, is dealt with. Similarly the psychological integration which makes up the psychical aspect. Next it seems profitable to discuss the contributions of the psycho-analytic

* A tropism is an inherent tendency to be attracted or repelled by a given stimulus. These are most clearly seen in unicellular organisms, but may also be exemplified by the tendency of a flower to turn towards the sunlight.

† Conditioned reflexes are explained in Chapter II.

schools, who have done much to throw light on the inter-relationships of various physical and mental environmental factors, which contribute towards the total personality, and consider their applicability and limitations. Further sidelights on these inter-relationships are afforded by brief discussion of certain abnormal personalities. Finally the spiritual aspect of Personality is discussed, wherein it becomes fully organized and significant. Again, let it be emphasized that our central thesis is, that however much we study, however much we analyse any personality, he remains one, indivisible and unique.

CHAPTER II

THE RELATIONSHIP OF BODY AND MIND

ACCORDING to the definition proposed in the last chapter, the term Personality signifies the total mental and bodily constitution of a human being, at all stages of development, both in relation to himself and to his environment. In setting out to study Personality as a whole, it is essential to formulate a definite concept as to the relationship of Body and Mind. Many theories have been advanced to this end, but an attempt to prove the truth of the particular hypothesis adopted is beyond the scope of a work such as this. Indeed it is a task which is as futile as it is difficult. In Chapter X there will be occasion to notice in what different ways individuals react in their thoughts and feelings to events, theories and objects; and how impossible it is for those of different types to appreciate each other's point of view. Moreover, we must recognize that there is considerable variation in such reactions, even in the same individual, at different periods of life. Such being the case, it is inevitable that there must be differences in the way in which the relationship of Body and Mind appeals to the various types of persons.

In the present state of our knowledge, our appreciation of the facts is all too imperfect, and, with no absolute standard in this respect, any theory must be open to criticism. Each will follow the presentation which attracts him, and all that can be done is to accept some definite conception of the problem on one hypothesis or other and use it to explain our observations as best it may.

It was during the seventeenth and eighteenth centuries that this question first came to be seriously discussed, in all its bearings, by philosophers of the Christian era. The Greeks had dealt with this fundamental problem according to their lights, while the schoolmen had taken an animistic standpoint as a matter of course; but both were chiefly concerned with the ethical aspect of the problem, as has already been pointed out. During these centuries, six great philosophers were found to champion the six possible ways of dealing with the relationship.[1]

First in chronological order, comes the animistic dualism of Descartes, who distinguished sharply between the extended material substance of body and the unextended immaterial substance of soul. He considers the body to be entirely mechanical, while the soul, the thinking rational ego, is a separate creation which acts on the body and is acted on by it, during the life of the body, with causal relationship between them. But since the soul is unextended, it cannot be destroyed and so is immortal. Mind and Body, therefore, are two separate creations, and in spite of their interaction, are essentially distinct.

Secondly, there was the parallelistic animism of Leibnitz, who held that body and soul are two separate entities, entirely independent, but always acting in relationship, because of the pre-established harmony of their nature invested in them by God at the moment of their creation. As he described it, Body and Soul are like two chronometers which, having been started together, always keep in time with each other, in virtue of their essential accuracy.

Thirdly, we have the identity hypothesis of Spinoza, who considered Body and Mind as identical but presenting two aspects for examination, one physical and the other psychical. Thus, we might consider the time registered by a chronometer from the visual standpoint, by looking at its face, or from the auditory standpoint by listening to its chime.

Fourthly, there was the thoroughgoing materialism of Hobbes, who described everything in terms of Body and Motion, and regarded the soul as a figment of the imagination.

In contrast to this, was the fifth view, that of Berkeley, who denied the reality of everything except the soul, holding that material things had no existence whatever, apart from their presentation to the soul. He based his argument, on the fact that the only evidence he had of these material things was through his senses, and, inasmuch as the senses are an attribute of the soul, there is no reality but the soul.

This led to the sixth and last possible thesis, the complete scepticism of Hume. He agreed with Berkeley as to the absence of reliable evidence of material things, but pointed out that there was no more reliable evidence for the soul. He was therefore led to the view that both Body and Soul are fictitious.

Kant attempted to strike a balance, between several of these hypotheses, especially the last two, by postulating two realms of reality. Firstly, the empirical reality or reality of experience, which comprises all material objects, including the body and the concepts of space and time. All phenomena pertaining to this realm were only real in so far as they were known to the soul, which itself belonged to a higher realm of reality, independent of space and time.

From these theses have originated the more recent doctrines, which have sought to explain the relationship we are considering. Animism, essentially dualistic, insists that some outside power intervenes in the ordered evolution of material things, especially at such points as the origin of life and of mental activity, and that this intervention must be presumed if these phenomena are to be adequately explained. This theory lost ground on the whole, in spite of the rather mixed support given to it by James,[2] till it gained a new lease of life from the brilliant philosophical *tour de force* of Bergson.[3] Of recent years however, in spite of the advocacy of McDougall,[1] it does not receive so much support from philosophers as formerly. Of the parallelistic doctrines founded on the teaching of Leibnitz, strict epiphenomenalism and psycho-physical parallelism, find few adherents. On the other hand, some form of derivative of the identity-hypothesis of Spinoza would seem to find increasing favour in the eyes of the scientific and philosophic world. This is largely due to the work of Huxley,[4] who insisted on the principle that there is no psychosis without a neurosis. That is to say, that every mental process is accompanied by, and is a function of the activity of nervous structure, arranged in greater or less complexity.

At first sight, common sense seems to tell us that immaterial mind cannot be identical with material body, but this idea of strict correlation between, and essential identity of Mind and Body, has become more easy to accept, in view of the advances in physical science which have taken place in the last 25 years. These have tended to show that material mass is less fundamental than was supposed, and that such concepts as energy and matter are not so different as at first sight appears. These researches have led natural philosophers back to the doctrine of Spinoza, which is the standpoint adopted in this presentation of personality. Metaphysical argument has no place in a naturalistic scheme, but it is suggested that, as Holt[5] and Russell[6] have pointed out, the conceptions of mental and bodily substance, of mind stuff and body stuff, are misleading. What we are concerned with is a common process involving the function of certain anatomical structures. On the one hand, this function may be studied according to psychological laws, and in so doing we examine the psychoses in Huxley's sense. On the other hand, this function may be examined according to physiological laws, when we observe the neuroses in the same connotation. As to what it is that characterizes mind as opposed to matter, or, to state the same problem in other terms, how is psychology to be distinguished from physics, Mr. Bertrand Russell[6] gives the answer, that psychology and physics are distinguished by the nature of their causal laws, and not by their subject-matter. Seeking to find what constitutes mind, Mr. Russell rejects consciousness, the power of acquiring experience, and memory, as characteristic of mental activity, because none of them are broad enough to comprise the whole. He suggests that subjectivity is a characteristic which more approximately satisfies the requirements of the definition. Those particulars which constitute the physical world can be collected into sets, in two different ways. One of these makes a bundle of all those particulars, that are appearances of a given thing from different places. This is the objective view, and the "given thing" is treated as an object, and studied according to physical laws, which deal with its weight, its colour, its hardness, etc. The other makes a bundle of all those particulars which are appearances of different things from a given place. A bundle of this latter sort, at a given time, is called a perspective; taken throughout a period of time, it is called a biography, and the "given thing" in this case is a subject to be studied according to psychological laws, which may describe its feelings, its cognitions, etc. Subjectivity is the characteristic of perspectives and biographies, the characteristic of giving the view of the world from a certain place. Subjectivity is not in itself a sufficient definition of Mind, since perspectives and biographies do not necessarily involve consciousness, experience, memory and the other characteristics of mental phenomena which are much more than mere subjectivity. But subjectivity is an essential in the definition of Mind, for this is the aspect of "things" with which psychology has to deal.

As has been said above, matter as usually understood is only a "logical fiction", invented because it gives a convenient method of stating causal law. But matter, as we know it, is inferred from its appearances; and although, according to certain metaphysicians, these appearances are of the same sort in ultimate analysis as are those from which the psychologist infers his data, yet, for physics the aspect is the objective one. The physicist is concerned with how his "piece of matter" looks, from every point of view, and by the comparison of these view-points, he verifies his physical laws and defines his matter. The causal laws of physics differ from those of psychology, in that they connect a particular aspect of the same piece of matter with its other appearances, instead of connecting several pieces of matter with each other in the same perspective. For example, suppose I stand in a room containing a chair, a table, a desk and a couch, the psychical aspect of this arrangement of "Me" is how the chair, table, desk and couch appear to me. The physical aspect of Me is how I appear from the chair, table, desk and couch, respectively. From this it follows that mental processes comprise functioning of the organism, arranged and integrated, from the subjective standpoint according to psychical laws; while bodily phenomena are the same functions arranged and integrated from the objective standpoint according to physical laws. Thus John Brown is walking along a path. Suppose first, that I am Tom Smith minutely observing John Brown. I may describe the action of his muscles, which are involved in the rhythmical movements of his legs, arms and body, the secretion of his various glands, the rate of his pulse and respiration, and so on, according to the means at my disposal for accurate observation. Such is the attitude of the extreme behaviourist who treats John Brown as an object, and neglects any question of consciousness on the part of the latter as uninteresting, since it cannot be observed and recorded. But all these records and observations are physiological and not psychological. But now suppose, that I am not Tom Smith, but am John Brown, then my observations may be quite different. I take the subjective attitude, and cease to be interested in excursions of muscles and secretions of glands, but am concerned with feelings of pleasure or otherwise, depending on perceptions of heat or fatigue, with images of former walks, with perceptions of present objects, and perhaps with prospective images of the end of the walk. This is the attitude of the introspective psychologist whose records are essentially psychological. However, as Koffka[7] has pointed out, introspection alone cannot be adequate for two reasons. Firstly, there is no criterion that the observations of introspection are correct, since any two persons may not describe the subjective experience of an object, even such as a primary colour, in the same terms. Secondly, only those mental processes which are "in the focus of attention" can be examined introspectively, and this limits and distorts the mental content to an unwarrantable extent. Nor is "strict behaviourism" in better case. All it can do, if it remains true to its own principles, which fortunately it has never done, is to learn new special facts about the physiology of the muscles and the glands. And, again, this method demands a specific attitude of the observer. He is not to trust to his first impression, which lets him see a clever dog searching for a hidden piece of food, or the slow deliberating glance of a chimpanzee, wanting a banana out of his reach. He does not see rage or fear or joy, but only movements of limbs and secretions. To get over these limitations of the two attitudes we must regard any situation as a whole, and realize that, when we try to analyse, we destroy the significance of the whole. John Brown's walk is only significant when both his muscular actions and his subjective experiences are taken into account, and to divorce one from the other is to destroy the significance of the walk. As Semon[8] pointed out, if we allow that behaviour is a response to stimuli, the nature of that response is determined by the structural organization of the organism, and this structural organization, he termed an engram. Any given engram owes its form partly to heredity, that is to inherent constitution dependent on mnemic influences* on the germ-plasm;

* By mnemic influences we mean lasting modifications impressed on the organism as a result of activation on some previous occasion.

partly to previous environmental influences, that is, to mnemic influences on the neuro-muscular and glandular systems; and partly to the effect of the present stimuli, none of which can have significance except in virtue of their relationship with the other two. We may say then, that any behaviour is the result of activation of an engram. When such an engram is activated, certain results ensue. When examined objectively, we describe muscular contractions and glandular secretions. When examined subjectively, we describe cognitions or reception of impressions, affects or feelings, and conations or impulses to action. Thus we may take the same process of activation and describe it in terms of physiology, or in terms of psychology, but we are, in fact, talking of different aspects of the same process. Moreover, that process must be considered as a whole in all its aspects, if it is to retain its full significance. John Brown is walking along a path in virtue of a complicated engram established in his neuromuscular system, and he walks in the way he does in virtue of the organization of that engram. If this organization was altered, his behaviour would be altered, and he might run or walk backwards; and in that case different objective physiological observations would be recorded by Tom Smith, and different subjective psychological experiences would be recorded by John Brown.

This distinction between subjectivity and objectivity, as characteristic of mental and physical respectively, has been stated in another way by Lloyd Morgan.[9] He distinguishes the "ings" from the "eds." All that constitutes minding is mental, but everything that is minded is physical. Similarly, all that is concerned with remembering is mental, and all that is remembered is physical, and so with hearing and heard and the rest. Lloyd Morgan would not, of course, deny that the things minded exist in mind, and it may be argued, going back to Berkeley, that there is no proof that that which is minded exists outside what Mr. Russell would call the biography of the individual who is minding. Yet it is pragmatically useful to regard those things which are minded as having an independent material existence "out there" in space and time. If we accept this position we must always remember that there is, in the complex relationship between the minding and the minded, what Lloyd Morgan terms an advenient physical influence from the material object, and a projicient psychical reference from our own minds, which, together with intervenient influences from the environment and ourselves, go to make up the complex of how we mind the things minded. For example, appreciation of a sunset depends on the advenient influence of the light waves on the retina—the sensitive portion of the eye; on the projicient reference, out there in the sky; of the effect of these light waves on our nervous system; together with the intervenient influence of various factors from the environment, such as the refraction of the atmosphere, and of other factors from ourselves such as the influence of association with images of previous sunsets. This complex constitutes an entity of which the sunset is the physical aspect and the subject's appreciation of the sunset is the psychical aspect. The latter is only significant when the whole complex is taken into account. So, if we apply this distinction, substituting bodily reactions of muscles and glands for separate entities "out in space," we arrive at the physiological reactions as things minded and the psychological reactions as the minding.

At this point to avoid confusion, we must distinguish clearly what we mean by Mind and Mental. These words have at least two connotations. The first will represent an activation of engrams, which have reached a certain complexity, considered from the subjective aspect and according to psychological laws of engraphic activity. The limits of this order will be found to vary according to the views of different authorities; for to some, mental phenomena are synonymous with conscious phenomena, while to others the term mental comprises a great deal more. However, in general, when people talk of certain phenomena being in mind they mean that these phenomena are dependent on the activation of engrams of a certain complexity of organization. The subjective aspect of that activity involves experiences whose upper limit is full consciousness, and whose lower limit is ill defined and varying, but which has its place somewhere above the order of purely reflex phenomena.

The second connotation which is given to the word mental is of much wider significance. This is the psychological aspect of any engram, however simple. This use of the word mental corresponds to the subjectivity of Russell, and to the psychosis of Huxley. In the lower orders of the hierarchy of mental processes, this aspect is not obvious, and cannot be appreciated by introspection. Yet we must accept the fact that it exists. If we are to be strict correlationists we must allow that if there is no psychosis without a neurosis, then there is no neurosis without a psychosis, and even the simple spinal reflex must have a mental correlate of some sort. However, as this is so far below the level of consciousness, we can have no idea of its nature. As for the individual, so also for the species. In this sense of the word we must admit mental phenomena, not only in man and the higher animals, but also in the lower animals down to the very simplest forms of life. Some have even sought to extend the parallel to inanimate objects, though this is stretching the connotation beyond a point where it is pragmatically useful.

Our standpoint in this study of personality is to be one of strict correlation. Every mental process however complicated, however abstract, is correlated with an activation of certain nerve cells, and of certain muscles and glands. Every activation of a group of neurones, however simple, is correlated with a mental reaction. One aspect of such an activation is the mental aspect, and is described in terms of experience, though this experience need not be conscious. The other aspect is bodily, and is described in terms of activity either of glands or muscles, together with biochemical and electrical changes in the neurones themselves. These aspects may not be equally obvious, either to the subject himself or to the observer. Take as instances purposive activity, feeling and thought. In the first, the physiological aspect of muscular activity is obvious both to the subject and to the observer. No mental aspect can be obvious to the observer, and is therefore of little account to the strict behaviourist. None the less such mental aspect exists and can be detected by introspection. In purposive activity, the observer sees the movements and the effects of the movements of the striped muscles, and may be able to detect various glandular activities, and the electrical changes which are induced by activation of the neurone. The subject also sees this movement, but the conation, the setting towards and carrying out of these movements, is present as a definite and generally quite conscious mental phenomenon which is an essential part of the whole complex. So in feeling, the bodily activity takes the form of secretion of glands and contraction of unstriped muscles which can be detected by the observer, by special methods, though less readily than in the case of purposive activity. The mental activity takes the form of feeling, whether in the primitive form of the pleasure-unpleasure relationship, or in the form of the more complex derivatives, the simple and compound emotions. Thought has also these two aspects; the mental aspect is obvious by introspection, but the bodily aspect is much more difficult to detect. However, even in the case of thought, there is much evidence to support the view that appreciable bodily activity does take place. This consists of slight movements whether in the striped or unstriped muscles, and possibly also some secretory activity of glands. In addition to this there are the electrical changes in the neurones themselves which are demonstrable in all these processes.

As the essential basis, determining the production of both mental experience and bodily activity, we postulated the activation of systems of neurones grouped as engrams, and it is necessary to return to this concept and define it further. By the word engram, Semon[8] denotes "the permanent change wrought by a stimulus on the irritable tissue of the organism." The irritable tissue with which we are concerned at present, is that of the nervous system. What happens when a stimulus is applied to a sense organ may be illustrated by the following example. If light waves impinge upon the retina, they produce certain biochemical changes in the specialized cells which are sensitive to light, and which are termed rods and cones. As a result of these biochemical changes, activity proceeds along the optic nerve. This activity can be demonstrated as a difference of electric potential, spreading along the nerve. Still, though we can demonstrate this activation as an electrical energy change, it does not necessarily follow that the actual form of energy transmission is electrical. As Myers[10] has pointed out, the demonstrable form may not be identical with the actual form of energy, for there may be some higher type of energy, which we do not yet understand. The activity having reached the synapses, or points of contact between the separate nerve cells or neurones it will traverse a more or less complicated series of neurones to emerge finally in a common motor path, such as Sherrington[11] has described. (See opposite page.)

Thus a simple engram may involve nothing more than the blinking of the eyes in response to the flash of light. But the pattern of neurones so traversed by the activation, will depend on various factors and the engram may become

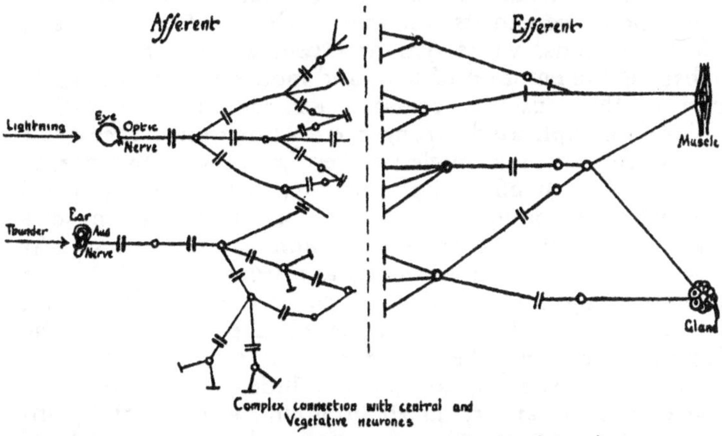

The whole comprises an engram whose activation determines a specific behaviour response

very complex. For instance, the response of the neurones in the visual system which are activated as a result of the retinal stimulation, may be integrated with the response of neurones whose activation proceeds from other receptors if these normally respond to specific stimuli, associated in the same stimulus pattern. This integration may be sufficiently complex to involve a conscious experience, or a perception; and the response may be likewise complicated, so as to involve movements of all the limbs for a prolonged period. For example, suppose that the light stimulus referred to has been afforded by a flash of lightning, then immediately afterwards there will occur as a rule an auditory stimulus of thunder. The ocular stimulus of the lightning and the auditory stimulus of the thunder may be said to belong to the same pattern of stimuli, so that they will be associated together, and an engram will be formed involving perception of a thunder storm, perhaps fear or awe, and perhaps complicated behaviour with the object of seeking shelter. The mental and physical response to these stimuli, thus associated, may be induced in the presence of one only; so that if lightning is seen, thunder will be inferred, even if it does not occur, and behaviour appropriate to lightning and thunder will ensue. Thus, on the supposition that the reaction induced on first seeing lightning and hearing thunder, was to experience fear and to run and hide, an engram has been established involving the optic nerve and its connexions, the auditory nerve and its connexions, vegetative and central neurones, which subserve the emotion of fear, and motor nerves, setting in motion the muscles necessary for running and hiding. All this complicated arrangement of neurones becomes a unity, and acts as a whole; either lightning or thunder, or both, will set it off, and the activity will always proceed through the common motor path involving the muscles which induce the movements of running and hiding. At the same time other activities are aroused which induce the sweating and shaking which accompany fear. But in addition to all this, is a mental aspect of seeing the lightning, hearing the thunder, feeling the fear and the impulse and striving to run and hide. So we see that the engram is an organized grouping, whose activity involves physical phenomena on the one hand, and psychical activity on the other. Similarly, the visual stimulus of a small tabby animal, the auditory stimulus of a purr, the tactile stimulus of soft fur, and perhaps a less pleasing olfactory stimulus, belong to the same pattern of stimuli. The activation of neurones started by any of these various stimuli are eventually grouped together, and from the psychical aspect a mental response emerges, which is symbolized by the name cat, and this may involve actions of stroking or kicking as the case may be.

How these stimuli come to be associated into such patterns, and how the systems of neurones activated by them are integrated into a definite engram, can be understood by reference to the law of the conditioned response which will be fully described in Chapter IV. The researches of Pawlow[12] demonstrated the nature of the conditioned reflex response. To take a very simple case as an illustration. He noted the production of salivation in a dog on being shown food. Eventually he found that the stimulus induced by the ringing of a bell had been so associated with food that salivation ensued directly the bell was rung, even in the absence of food. This showed that when one stimulus is continually associated with another, the activations of the corresponding neurones become integrated, and pass over to the efferent side, to issue by the same motor path, whichever stimulus starts the activation. Such a grouping of neurones so that they react together, represents a permanent influence on the irritable nervous tissue, and this type of neurone complex, as has been said, is called an engram by Semon. Such engrams may be simple or extremely complex. This complexity may be arrived at by the gathering in of other engrams, which are correlated with associated cognitions, affects or conations. Moreover it is maintained, that however complex an engram may be, its constitution may be explained on the basis of the conditioned response. McDougall[13] pours scorn on the idea that complicated mental processes can be analysed into conditioned responses ; and to say that an abstract mathematical concept is nothing but a conditioned response, does seem absurd on the face of it. An attempt will be made in Chapters IV, V, and VI to trace the connexion existing between the simple reflex, only describable from the physical aspect, and the more complex mental responses, which can only be described from the psychical aspect. It is suggested that the principle of emergence, to be dealt with in the next Chapter, will do something to remove McDougall's difficulty.

These engrams, once established, are subject to change in the course of life. They may be reintegrated or disintegrated, and their constitution and history has been thus expressed by Semon, in what he terms his Mnemic laws. "All simultaneous excitations within an organism form a coherent simultaneous excitation-complex, which acts engraphically, that is it leaves behind it a coherent engram-complex, constituting a definite unit," such as that described above for the lightning-thunder pattern. That is to say, when two or more systems of neurones are activated together, according to any of the types of association familiar to the psychologists, a new and more or less permanent grouping will result. The partial recurrence of the excitation-complex, which left behind it a simultaneous engram-complex, acts ecphorically on the latter, whether the recurrence be in the form of original or mnemic excitations. By acting ecphorically we mean, that any one stimulus results in the activation of the whole engram. For example, the hearing of a purr, or even the memory of a purr brings up into consciousness the whole complex cat. " Association depends on the conjunction of single engrams; it makes its appearance during their relatively isolated activation and originates simply from the presence of the respective components in the same simultaneous complex. From this it follows, that if a new stimulus arises which is similar to the original stimulus, the new group of neurones so activated, and the old group which has already formed an engram, will tend to be activated as a whole and result in the formation of a more complex engram."

We may picture the growth of personality on the basis of increasing complexities of engrams, which become integrated and associated, in the way which Sherrington has shown to be typical of the nervous system. This applies both to the individual and to the species. In the individual, to begin with, the arrangement of neurones is simple, chiefly on the basis of the reflex response. Soon, with the continual conditioning of these responses, more complicated engrams are successively formed, which have, for the mental aspect of their response, the more complicated phenomena of ideation and emotion, sentiments and beliefs and so on, which we shall have occasion to examine at a later stage, and for their bodily aspect, various complicated muscular and glandular responses. So with the species, in the lower animal the arrangements of neurones are simple in the extreme, but with the rise in evolutionary complexity, they group themselves into more and more complex engrams, till in man, with a great increase of nervous tissue, they become extremely complicated.

As has been said already, however complex, or however simple an engram may be, two manifestations present themselves for description as a result of its activation. A subjective mental activity will be experienced, and if at the conscious level, can be detected and described by introspection; and even if below this level, it may be investigated by special methods such as hypnosis. Also an objective physical behaviour can be detected by an observer, as the second aspect of the process. This difference of aspect in recording the activation of an engram is the difference between body and mind, so that, while for descriptive purposes they are different, they are essentially the same thing. We therefore accept the metaphysical standpoint, which makes no distinction between Body and

Mind except in respect of the causal laws, by which we explain the phenomena observed, in each sphere respectively. We take as a basis of both, the activation of groups of neurones, and describe the mental phenomena which ensue, according to psychological laws, and the bodily phenomena, which may be observed, according to physiological laws. Our next task must be to discuss how, in the course of this increasing evolutionary complexity, new forms arise, whether bodily or mental.

CHAPTER III

THE PRINCIPLE OF EMERGENCE

IN our consideration of personality, it will be necessary to study the bodily and mental components which go to make up the whole, and it is very necessary to make quite clear how the synthesis from the simple to the complex takes place. As has been noted in the last Chapter, the statement that any complex process is nothing but such and such simpler components, into which it can be analysed, is neither accurate nor even plausible. The same difficulty applies to any synthetic conception, and one of the features of Darwinism which failed to bring conviction, was that evolutionary progress could emanate from nothing but infinitesimal variations. This original concept of evolution is no longer acceptable, and nature does not seem to proceed in that smooth course, but rather by a series of leaps and bounds. As Lloyd Morgan [1] says, " The orderly sequence of evolution, historically viewed, appears to present from time to time, something genuinely new. Salient examples are afforded in the advent of life, in the advent of mind, and in the advent of reflective thought." In the study of personality this conception of emergence is of great importance.

Let us take a simple example from the realm of chemistry. Under certain environmental conditions, Hydrogen and Oxygen combine to form the compound water. This water is a new emergent, it has no resemblance either to Hydrogen or Oxygen, but is a fresh entity of itself. It is not true to say, that water is nothing but Hydrogen and Oxygen. Yet water involves these two elements; and in the absence of either of them it cannot exist. If water is not only Hydrogen and Oxygen, something else must be involved in its production. This something else is a special relatedness of the component elements to each other and to the environment. Hydrogen and Oxygen can be mixed in all sorts of ways, subjected to all sorts of influences from the environment, thermal, electrical, etc.; but unless and until the requisite specific relatedness is achieved, there is no integration of the elements into water. Further, water does not disintegrate into its components, except in special conditions of the environment, because under the above circumstances the molecules are arranged in a new form or structure which is inherently stable. This special relatedness is the secret of new emergence, and goes far to overcome the difficulty of the 'nothing but' hypothesis. The causal agency which brings about the special relatedness is a metaphysical question which does not concern us here. That it happens is all that we need to know, and whether brought about by an intervenient Deity, by the laws of the universe, or what not, is no concern of ours.

It is advisable to trace the process of emergence throughout evolution, to supplement our study of body-mind relationship, and to support the thesis that all phenomena, mental and physical, evolve without the intervention of any outside agency, from the simplest to the most complex. For the sake of clarity, however, it is as well not to go back beyond the modern physical conception of the atom, for such units as Alexander's[2] space-time elements are hard to grasp and are necessarily speculative. Physicists have shown that the atom consists of systems of protons and electrons, that is of positive and negative electrical charges, in relation to each other. This is true for all atoms, and brings out the importance of relatedness, more than any other example could. Gold and Oxygen are both composed of protons and electrons, differing only in their relation to each other. Hence this relatedness is the variable factor in the composition of these utterly different elements. The same is true of the combination of atoms into molecules in respect of the importance of relatedness in determining differences. Thus, given different forms of relatedness and different environmental conditions, the combination of the same component atoms may result in different emergents. For instance, to return to the combination of hydrogen and oxygen; under certain conditions, water emerges, but under other conditions hydrogen peroxide emerges. This is a substance entirely different, not only from the component elements, but also from the other emergent, water. This difference is due, not only to the quantitative proportion of atoms in the molecules, but also to the structural form taken by the molecule. In the organic chemical compounds this variation in emergents from the same elements is still more noticeable, for the varieties of carbon, hydrogen, oxygen and nitrogen combinations are legion. Indeed, carbon by itself is capable of the most various manifestations depending on the relatedness of its atoms. Molecular structure seems to be chiefly responsible for the properties of substances, and this is best exemplified by the various types of crystals, which are dependent on the form taken in the arrangement of the atoms within the molecules. It was the discovery of the significance of "form" in molecular structure, that led to the greatest advances in chemistry, the realization of the importance of the ring form in the benzine group being, perhaps, the best known and most fruitful of such advances. So far we may have a clear idea of the environmental conditions, and the special relatedness which determine the emergence of the new entity; but at the next stage, that of the emergence of life from the organic chemical compounds, this factor is beyond our knowledge. It is at this point, above all others, that the animists claim that all the rival philosophical theories have failed. They say that it is absolutely necessary to postulate an influence coming in from outside, to induce this absolute change between living and dead tissue, which completely evades all our attempts at discovery. This argument, however, only seems to obscure the issue still further. In formulating our explanations of any problem, there is considerable pragmatic sanction for postulating that all concepts, scientific and philosophical, should be as simple as possible, should be expressed in terms of the known rather than the unknown, should work along the lines of laws already established, rather than by the manufacture of new laws. After all, the laws which have served us to understand what we know of the structure of the universe, are relatively simple and relatively few. The advances which have been made have been rather in the nature of amplifications and fresh orientations of the old laws, than of complete refutations of them; witness the relationship between Newton and Einstein, in their conception of the universe. The apparent complete change of outlook introduced by the latter does not depend on the total abandonment of any of Newton's principles, but rather on a new orientation. The animistic concept of something coming in anew, from the outside, leaves much unexplained. For example, what exactly is this new thing and where is this outside and what resides there. It seems more reasonable to postulate that the new thing is the special relatedness, and that that makes the difference between protoplasm dead and protoplasm alive. Because we do not know what this relatedness is, it does not follow that we shall never know it. Moreover, it is quite possible that although this special relatedness is potentially knowable, actually it is unknowable, because the requisite conditions of environment can never be artificially produced on this earth. It is suggested that the animistic doctrine of an influence coming from outside is less valuable as a concept to explain the origin of life than the doctrine of life as an emergent, depending on an unknown relatedness, at least analogous to other forms of relatedness which, we have seen, are necessary for the emergence of new entities. If the exact relatedness which constitutes the difference between living and dead protoplasm still escapes us, recent work on cellular physiology and chemistry does point the way for further research. For example, Lillie[3] remarks that "it is a peculiarity of living matter, as distinguished from non-living matter, that it is never found in a diffuse, unorganized or formless state, but always composing definite individualized systems or organisms." It may not be true to say that life cannot exist independently of cellular structure and organization, but this structural form exerts a profound influence on life. Not only this, but the various proteins which make up the protoplasm of various species present definite composition and stereo-chemical configuration, which differentiates them from the proteins of other species, suggesting that the variations in life activity, and hereditary characteristics of different species, depend on variations in the molecular structure of their protoplasm. This is analogous to the variations in crystalline form, and although proteins are colloidal, under certain conditions crystals of these compounds may be produced. Thus working with the hæmoglobin of various species, Reichart and Brown[4] have shown that the crystals produced are morphologically distinct. This principle of molecular structure is, therefore, likely to comprise the important factor in the special relatedness we call life. As Lillie says "living systems are highly special developments; they represent a higher order of synthesis, and it is to be expected, that they should exhibit properties and activities which are absent in non-living systems. Hence the existence of a sharp contrast between the livingand the non-living—i.e., between organism and environment—is not in itself surprising. We know, however, that continuous transitions from the one to the other have existed and still exist; life has evolved from non-living matter in the past; and in the present, every living organism is the seat of a continual transformation of non-living into living matter. The chief problem of general physiology, is to trace the steps of this transition; i.e., to determine the nature of the synthesis by which the living matter, protoplasm, is built up from the non-living material, which it incorporates from the surroundings. Living organisms may be distinguished from dead organisms by several characteristic processes—metabolism, growth, automatic self-maintenance, reproduction and heredity, irritability, regulation and adaptation, and spontaneous activity. Metabolism is the constant chemical activity of living structure, whereby substances are continuously being broken down and rebuilt by a series of chemical changes which never cease. The rebuilding series of changes constitute the nutritive function of the organism, while the breaking-down series constitute its energy yielding function. These chemical changes are by no means all peculiar to organisms, though some only occur under the special relatedness which involves life. One of the consequences of constructive metabolism is growth. This is a definitely specific process, whereby new substance is built up to replace outworn or lost substance, or a general increase in size of the organism is attained. Again, a specialized part of the organism may be separated from the parent, to grow into a new organism. Whether the growth be individual for the purpose of self-maintenance, or reproductive, the new tissue is built up on the same plan as the old. This may be due to the specific molecular form, which we have seen to be characteristic of different species. If this specificity of molecular form could be proved, it would explain many of the problems of heredity more satisfactorily than can be done at present.

Irritability is the characteristic of living organisms, whereby they respond to changes in the environment (stimuli) by changes in themselves (response). This means that the processes of metabolism are capable of modification by slight changes in the environmental media, a phenomenon not confined to living organisms. However, with the higher degrees of relatedness, this irritability becomes regulated and adapted, and in this way the organism becomes better and better adjusted to the environment. By adaptation the reciprocal relations of stimulus and response are so organized, that the species is enabled to survive. Further, this adaptation and organization proceeds, not only between the organism and its environment, but also within the organism itself by the process known as integration. By this means the animal is enabled to act as a whole, and the structural form of the organization is so adapted to the environment that spontaneous activities, directed to some definite end, become possible.

Life having once emerged, the process of evolution goes on by the emergence of new qualities, whose components can be studied without great difficulty, and the laws of whose relatedness, and the environmental conditions necessary for whose existence, have in large measure been worked out. A differing relatedness of very similar constituents determines the distinction between plant and animal, the one characterized by a dominant vegetative function, and the other by a dominant motor function.

In our present study we are concerned with the animal kingdom, and especially the emergence of the nervous system. This system would seem to be evolved from a gradual specialization of certain functions, characteristic of living protoplasm. These are the negative and positive tropisms, met with in the lowest forms of living organisms such as the Amœba. Certain mechanical thermal and electrical stimuli, applied to such living protoplasm, induce motion of the whole organism towards the source of these stimuli. Other stimuli of a different mode, or different intensity, result in the motion of the whole organism away from the source of the stimulus. These processes are chiefly of a chemical nature at this stage of existence. When the stage of the unicellular organism has been passed the cellular organization of protoplasmic structure modifies its reaction to a remarkable extent. Division of labour and differentiation of function are the chief characteristics of further growth. The researches of Parker[5] and others, on the elementary types of nervous reaction, demonstrate how the neuromuscular system is developed in the progress of evolution. In the sponges the earliest differentiation is towards contractile tissue, which is capable of direct response to stimuli without the intervention of tissue differentiated to subserve receptive and conductive function. In certain cœlenterates we find the next differentiation of a receptor cell in close contact with the effector cells. Then, between the outer and inner layers of cells—the ectoderm and the entoderm—there develops the nerve net. This is conductive tissue, which conveys activation from the point of stimulus all over the animal in any direction. In the higher cœlenterates some polarization of the nerve net is already met with, so that the activation is inhibited from passing in any direction, except by the one specific route from the receptor to the corresponding effector. From this polarization is derived the nerve fibre of the higher animals, which can only conduct in one direction. These nerve fibres and cells are then further differentiated so as to serve special functions, and concentrated in certain regions of the body. From this specialized structural arrangement are derived the central and peripheral nervous systems, characteristic of all animals higher in the evolutionary scale. As Sherrington[6] has shown, the nervous system gradually takes on the directive and integrative control of the whole body, so that every activity, of whatever nature, must be considered in relation to this system, and all activity, if not immediately initiated by it, is under nervous control. The primitive chemical activities are superseded so far as pre-eminence is concerned, but they persist as a reinforcing agent in the form of the endocrine system, to be studied in Chapter V. It does not follow from this that any given bodily function has no direct influence on another bodily function, without central nervous intervention, but it is mainly in relation to the elaboration and differential development of the nervous system, that evolutionary progress takes place. The basis from which this developmental progress is derived, is the reflex response. This response depends on certain differentiated structures in the body of the animal. Firstly, we get a specialized area of tissue, a receptor, which is sensitive to stimuli from the environment of the animal, or from other parts of its own body. These stimuli induce biochemical changes in this specialized tissue, resulting in a liberation of some form of energy, which is observed as a change in electrical potential. Secondly, we get a specially differentiated tissue whose function it is to conduct the activation induced by the response of the receptor. Thirdly, we get a specialized structure within the body, whose function it is to receive this afferent activation from one or more receptors, and distribute it to efferent conductive tissue, which forms the fourth link in the chain of the response. This conductive tissue conveys the activation to one or more end-organs, which determine the contraction of muscles or secretion of glands, the emergent from whose composite action constitutes the behaviour of the organism.

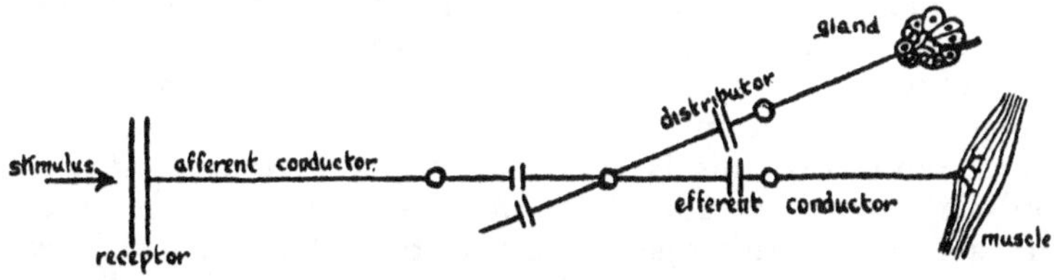

Such a description of the reflex response is incomplete, for even the simplest response involves not only the sequence described above, but also, as has been pointed out in Chapter II, a mental accompaniment, involving a low grade of cognition or awareness of stimulus and conation or striving for activity, along with affect or feeling, if any neurones of the vegetative nervous system are involved. The word mental is here used in the second of the two connotations, as described above. To describe the nature of the mental accompaniment of this response is impossible, so far is it below the level of conscious awareness. Hence the importance of using such technical terms as cognition, which does not necessarily involve awareness or imply consciousness. Indeed, this difficulty of appreciating these low level mental phenomena is a very serious handicap to psychology, especially as we have no everyday words in the language to describe them. They may be inferred, in a vague way, and modern psycho-pathology has shown that much which previously had seemed far below this level of conscious awareness is available for examination; but they cannot be observed with that precision which is possible with physical phenomena. The clearer understanding of the lower reflexes which have become suppressed, such as the mass reflex, has been of great assistance in the progress of neurology; but we are still groping in the dark for the suppressed and fused elements in the march of psychological evolution, and inference, which is all too probably erroneous, is all that we can use. For example, we may observe the amœba protrude its pseudopodia and engulf the diatom, and we must infer that this activity is accompanied by some sort of psychical experience, but what sort of low grade cognition and affect and conation this experience may be, must be a matter of pure conjecture.

The terms suppression and fusion which we owe to Rivers[7] are important, and require definition. By suppression is meant that an activity, which at one stage of evolution was useful in everyday life, has, with the march of progress, not only become useless but has ceased to make any obvious contribution to the total behaviour of the organism. An example of this is the mass reflex in man, which is only disclosed by complete division of the spinal cord. As a result of this operation, only the relatively low level nervous structure of the lumbo-sacral cord is able to function. Any stimulus applied to the lower limb causes defensive withdrawal of the limb by action of the flexor muscles, certain vasomotor changes, sweating and voiding of the bladder. In the healthy man there is no sign whatever of the existence of this reflex. It has been totally suppressed, but that such a defensive reaction may have been quite useful at some stage of animal evolution is obvious.

By fusion is meant that an activity, which has been useful and normal at one stage of evolution, is no longer dominant but still contributes to the total behaviour of the organism. A good example of this is the prespinal motor system in man, which, though dominated by the cortical motor system, still contributes to the tone of the muscular system. This is evident from the interference with muscular tonus and resultant power of posture and locomotion, which results from lesions destroying the functional activity of this system.

The next recognizable stage in the evolutionary process is the emergence of the conditioned reflex response from the combination of one or more reflexes, with fusion or suppression of certain of the component parts. These will be explained more fully in the next chapter and Pawlow's classical bell-ringing-salivation experiment has already been referred to. Experimental work has shown that many forms of behaviour may be explained in terms of the conditioned reflex. We must, however, guard against the suggestion that all sorts of behaviour are nothing but conditioned reflexes. The principle of emergence, with the advenience of something new depending on different relatedness, is essential. With the integration and elaboration of the conditioned reflex, there emerges the instinctive reaction. The word "instinct" has received so many connotations in these days of journalism, that a man is even said to have an instinct for salmon fishing. In this way it has almost lost its usefulness as a scientific term, but I use it in the sense originally applied to it by Lloyd Morgan.[8] A true instinctive response is one which is inherent in the disposition of the organism, and owes nothing to experience; such a response is seen in the swimming movements of the young duckling when put into water for the first time, or the pecking of the newly hatched chick at bright objects. Moreover, a true instinctive response is one which is not adapted to circumstances in the course of the animal's life, and is not modified by experience. Directly the behaviour of the animal is so adapted or modified, it is no longer purely instinctive. The loose use of this word "instinctive" has led to its extension both upwards and downwards in the scale. It is absurd, as has been said, to talk of an instinct for salmon fishing, but it is equally absurd to talk of the fission, and even the conjugation of unicellular animals as a reproductive instinct. It would seem more useful to retain the word "instinct" for a new emergent in evolutionary progress at a stage referred to by Lloyd Morgan as the advent of mind. This is one of the sudden advances which corresponds to that of the appearance of life lower in the scale, and the appearance of reflective thought at a higher level. Considered from the neurological aspect, reflex reactions are the function of a purely segmental nervous system, where there is no specialization between one segment and another. Instinctive reaction essentially depends on the specialization of certain segmental nervous structures to form a brain. This is a new departure in anatomical structure, and therefore it is only reasonable to expect a new departure in psychological reaction. Instinctive reaction will develop in intensity and potentiality with the increasing specialization and integration of the nervous system. This may reach a considerable degree of complexity in more than one type of nervous structure, as witnessed by the instinctive reactions of insects, whose neurological evolution takes a completely different form from that of vertebrates; but it should be noticed that in the case of insects there is remarkable rigidity of instinctive behaviour. The higher progress of evolution is in the direction of freedom of reaction, and with this comes the greater size and complexity of the brain tissue of vertebrates and finally the development of the cortex from the forebrain.

The exact neurological levels involved in instinctive action are extremely hard to determine. The so-called all-or-none * reaction of the instinct is generally supposed to be characteristic of thalamic behaviour, that is to say, the behaviour of an animal deprived of the cortical control exercised over the thalamus. Unfortunately, however, there is no zoological specimen which is normally "thalamic" † and so we cannot tell whether such an animal would exhibit pure instinctive reaction as here defined. Even the elasmobranch fishes have well-developed olfactory lobes, which are developments of the forebrain. Certain experiments of Sherrington on decerebrate dogs suggest that instinctive reaction involves cortical function, though this may be of a primitive type. Even such a universal instinctive action as the performance of the sexual act can only be carried out by the decerebrate dog if he is placed in position. He never goes to seek or initiate the act of his own accord. Such behaviour is reflex rather than fully instinctive; and there seems little doubt that instinct, as exhibited in the vertebrates, is dependent on some forebrain development. McDougall[9] has attempted to show that many activities, which previously have been regarded as purely instinctive, and therefore owing nothing to experience, such as nest-building in birds, are capable of modification and owe their fully developed form partly to adaptation. His examples are

* By "all-or-none" reaction is meant that if a response to stimulus is observed at all, that response is carried out at full intensity and with no grading either qualitative or quantitative.

† A "thalamic" animal would be one, whose nervous system was developed to the level of the basal ganglia: the structures which represent a stage in evolution, midway between the segmental nervous system, comprising spinal cord and brain stem, and the nervous system with a more or less developed forebrain or cortex.

hardly conclusive, and in many cases are definitely contradicted by the observations of experienced naturalists. For this reason, what McDougall calls the instincts of man would be better called by another name, for they do not come within this definition, though derived from and founded on instincts. They might be termed emotional dispositions. None the less, he is certainly right in insisting, that the behaviour of man is based on instinct and not on reason, as held by the older philosophers; but this is the sole justification for retaining the word "instinct," as applied to these higher emergents. It is at the level of instinctive response that the Mneme as described by Semon[10] becomes of importance for the psychologist. Semon's mnemic laws have already been referred to, and have to do with the influence of previous activation of the neurone paths involved in the present response. Our definition of instinctive response precludes any mnemic effect during the lifetime of the individual, but Semon postulated a mnemic effect on the germ plasm, as well as on the nervous system; and whether by the incidence of natural selection, or other selective influences, instinctive responses may well owe their nature to certain mnemic effects which have become manifest during the history of the race. It must be remembered, however, that although a previous activation of a pattern in germ plasm or nervous system exercises a profound influence on the result of a new activation, these two influences, the new and the old, enter into a special relatedness, and the resulting behaviour is a true emergent, with a unique character of its own. Directly we pass to the emergence of adapted behaviour, depending on new relatedness of instinctive types of behaviour, mnemic influence becomes of the greatest importance. Behaviour and mental experience in the broad sense, not only depend on the pattern of stimuli presented to the receptors, but on the engraphic effects of previous activations. Directly this factor comes in, we have a relationship of the present activity or experience to the past. Behaviour becomes linked up, one pattern of behaviour depending on another, and not appearing as an isolated phenomenon with no connexion with what has gone before. Mental phenomena, therefore, cannot be held to be static, but represent a stream, each item being indissolubly blended with what has gone before and what comes after. Considering the process from the psychical aspect, we must recognize a new relatedness of present sensation with images and the knowledge previously gained as a result of engraphic reactions. This results in the emergence of a perception, and the giving of meaning to the sensory impression. Such a perception is a quite definite new emergence, and is a structural totality which is appreciated as such, as the Gestalt theory has shown, and is not merely a bundle of images and sensations. This leads us to consciousness. This plane of consciousness and reflective thought involves a relatedness, which involves another definitely new emergence, such as that of life and mind. As with the case of instinct, this depends on a definite advance in the progress of structural evolution in the nervous system, namely, that of the full development of the forebrain into a definite cortical system of greater or less complexity. It is the function of the cortex which enables man to indulge in reflective thought, and so acquire his great ascendancy over the animals. As in the case of instinct, the complexity of conscious phenomena will depend on the complexity of brain structure, and it is not easy to define exactly what is conscious and what is not. Under these circumstances, it would not be correct to insist that the psychical aspect of all cortical function is conscious in the ordinary sense of the term. For example, dreams and somnambulisms certainly involve consciousness of a sort, and certainly involve cortical function, yet they are not usually referred to as conscious phenomena; and we have already seen that instinctive action involves some cortical function. Later we shall have occasion to examine in more detail these complexities of consciousness. An important feature of this level of emergence is that consciousness is characterized, amongst other things, by the property of continuance, as noted above. Here it is certainly no longer legitimate to talk of isolated occurrences, but only of a stream. Although it may be convenient to examine a cross section of this stream, it must be remembered that no unit in the stream has any significance except in relation to what has gone before, and to what is coming after. Certain upholders of animistic doctrines declare that their opponents fail because their explanations lose sight of this stream of consciousness. But in the present treatment of the problem, this difficulty does seem to be overcome, and an adequate explanation given of the waxing and waning of these processes. From both physical and psychical aspects, any process in consciousness may be described in three phases. Thus we have postulated that any mental process depends on the activation of an engram, or a series of neurones, determined in accordance with mnemic laws. This activation spreads from certain other neurones (the engram previously in action), reaches a maximum of intensity within the engram concerned, and passes away as the activation proceeds to another engram, viz., that successively in action. From the mental aspect, this process is experienced as a feeling of comingness, leading into a feeling of "passingawayness", as Lloyd Morgan has described it. Such a sequence results in a continuous stream of processes occurring in consciousness, and characteristic of it. This does not mean that such waxing and waning of activity in the engrams do not occur below the level of consciousness, but it is only at this level that there is sufficient integration of activity to give rise to the continuous stream of recognizable processes in which each event leans back towards the past and bends forward towards the future. As life emerges from matter as a new relatedness, whose exact nature and the conditions of environment requisite for whose appearance, are still shrouded in mystery, so consciousness emerges from life under conditions and with a relatedness which are only less obscure than those involved in the appearance of the latter. With full consciousness we have reached a plane in which the variation of relatedness of the individual is capable of enormous increase. At this plane we have possibilities of organized actions, organized feelings, and organized thought. From these emerged language, the step which, above all others, widens the radius of activity of mankind, when compared to the animals. Man ceases to be an individual, in the strictest sense, on the plane of life, for he cannot exist except in relation to his environment, and we cannot get a picture of his complete self, his personality, without taking into consideration that relationship. Directly we get to the plane of instinct, this radius of relatedness widens enormously. Sex, gregariousness, maternity, all bring him into closer, and at the same time, wider contact with others of his species, but it is only when language emerges, that the widest potentiality becomes apparent. Moreover the end is not yet. Man has not only acquired language and organized thought, but has freed his upper limbs from the duty of posture and locomotion. This has permitted all the advance in manipulative dexterity, which has meant so much in the march of progress. As knowledge has increased, so have the mechanical means of intercommunication, till we have arrived at the stage of aeroplanes and wireless telegraphy, with a promise for the future of a still greater expansion of man's radius of action. This means a greater and greater complexity of personality, which is indeed at present in a stage of instability due essentially to that rapidly increasing differentiation and growth.

But with this advance, which is making for new emergents, to what is the world progressing? Professor Alexander has described the goal as Deity, an emergent quality which is only so far being foreshadowed by what is best in human achievement. But with this future we are not concerned, except in so far as we postulate that the laws which direct man's progress in the evolutionary scheme are directed to a higher and better end, to harmony from chaos, and that we may therefore believe in the essential progress of humanity, in spite of apparent retrogressions.

In this scheme of emergent evolution, it is very important to notice, how the higher planes involve the lower planes. The atom cannot exist without the electrical charges whose special relatedness constitute that atom. The molecule cannot exist without atoms. Life is impossible without the phenomena belonging to the realms of chemistry and physics, and consciousness is inconceivable without life, and all that it involves. So at whatever level we are examining personality, we must remember that the particular type of relatedness we are concerned with involves all other forms of relatedness below it in the evolutionary scale. But it is not a mere summation of these, but a definite new entity of its own, different from its components and from everything else. This may be illustrated by a further reference to instinctive behaviour. All higher types of behaviour and especially human behaviour involve and are dependent on instinctive reactions, and not on higher "faculties" such as reason, memory, will and the like. But, inasmuch as in human behaviour these instinctive reactions have assumed a new relatedness, such behaviour is no longer pure instinct, but something else, which is instinctive but not instinct. Our chief concern will be with certain of the higher types of relatedness, discussed from the mental aspect, according to the laws of psychology, and with patterns of behaviour of the individual; and we must avoid the idea that the more complex processes are nothing but a combination of the less complex, and realize that they are something new, with a quality of their own. Another feature, which we noticed at the lower levels in the scale, operates also at the higher levels, and that is, that the same components do not always enter into the same relatedness to produce the same emergents. The importance of this is very great when we come to consider the patterns of behaviour of those who are abnormal, especially of the psycho-neurotics, but it also explains the differences between individual personalities. Behaviour depends on much the same components, whether we consider normal or abnormal individuals, but these differ in their relatedness, and so the emergents are quite distinct from each other. That the emergent behaviour depends on the integrity of nervous structure must be insisted upon and may be illustrated by the action of an anæsthetic. When the patient is waiting for the anæsthetist, he is behaving as a self-conscious reflective being. He thinks of himself in relation to the environment, and perhaps to the universe; he reflects on life and death, if he is of a philosophical turn of mind, or may merely be afraid he will choke. Then as he begins to breathe the gas, and his stream of thought becomes incoherent, he can no longer reason or reflect. He loses his grasp on the fact of his own existence, and loses that relatedness which involves reflection and self-consciousness. For the time being, he has ceased to exist as a being enjoying these functions. Next he loses all awareness, he is no longer a conscious person, all cortical function is abolished, as a result of the poisoning of the cortical cells. As the anæsthesia becomes deeper, various reflexes are lost and finally, if the poisoning is too intense, the molecular form involving life itself is disturbed and the patient dies. If the anæsthetising process stops short of this however, the poison gradually passes off, and with the recovery of cortical cells the functions of the patient recover "enjoyment" of the requisite relationships in an ascending scale, and awareness, self-consciousness, and reflection are in turn resumed.

This brings us to a position, in which it is possible to define more clearly, what is meant by personality.

Every personality is an emergent, and in virtue of its emergence, something quite new and quite distinct. Every personality is an emergent from a variety of components. These components group themselves into certain divisions which present themselves for study:

1. The various organs and systems of the body, and their respective functions. In view of its integrative and controlling function, the nervous system is by far the most important. The other organs and systems are chiefly of significance in the study of personality, in respect of their relation to this system, and in so far as they are modified by it and, in turn, modify its structure and function.

2. The component parts of the nervous system itself, especially the engraphic grouping of the neurones, and the response of these engrams to stimuli.

3. The mental correlates of these activations of engrams.

4. The relatedness of these mental and physical correlates with the environment, both in so far as the environment modifies them, and in so far as they modify the environment.

Further be it noted, that however similar these components may be in different personalities, their relatedness always varies, and therefore every personality is individual and is quite distinct from every other personality, just as every chemical compound is distinct from every other chemical compound. As we ascend in the evolutionary scale, the more complex is the pattern of unities in relation to each other, and the more subtle are the differences of the resultant product, even though these unities themselves are similar. Indeed, in dealing with human individuals, we might well reverse the adage and say,

"*Plus c'est la même chose plus ça change.*"

CHAPTER IV

THE ORGANIZATION OF BODILY FUNCTION

As has been said above, the whole of the body of the higher vertebrates is under the direction and control of the nervous system. Quite apart from the relationship of the body to the environment, the heart, lungs, digestive system and the rest, take their time from, and owe their activity to the action of this system, in such a way that the organization of bodily function entirely depends on it. Destruction of those nervous centres which are responsible for the regulation of these organs, seriously interferes with their action and, in the case of the heart and lungs, results in death. Similarly all activity of muscles, which are responsible for the movements of the body, depend on the influence of the nervous system and are entirely subservient to it. On the other hand, every activity of the muscles and internal organs results in the stimulus of nerves, whose business it is to convey messages back to the nervous centres. In this way there is a continuous interchange of messages and influences from nervous system to organs and from organs to nervous system, by the intervention of the peripheral nerves. At the same time, the various organs produce chemical substances which circulate in the blood and influence all other organs and especially the activity of the nervous system. With this question of "temperament" we shall deal in the next chapter. For the present, it is proposed to discuss the organization of the nervous system itself, since upon it depends the organization of the whole body. This system consists of a central part concerned with the reception and transmission of messages, analogous to the exchange in a telephone system, and of a peripheral part composed of the nerves which convey messages between the nervous system and the end organs. These nerves are analogous to the wires of the telephone. The end organs are the structures by means of which messages are received from the organs, or in the case of the special senses, from the environment, and transmitted to the central exchange, and are analogous to the instruments belonging to the various subscribers to the telephone system.

That part of the system which is concerned with receiving messages from the organs and transmitting them to the centres is the afferent part, while that concerned with transmission of messages from the centres to the organs is the efferent part.

The nervous system consists of two parts, the central nervous system proper and the vegetative system. These in turn are each divided into two parts. The vegetative system is made up of an autonomic and sympathetic system which are complementary to each other, and which, between them, organize all the functions of the body concerned with nutrition in the widest sense of the term. The central system is divided into a spinal part, including the brain-stem and the brain proper. Between them these organize both physical and psychical activity. The term brain-stem is applied to that part of the nervous system which, although included in the skull, functions in respect of the nerves of the face and head, in the same way as the spinal cord functions in relation to the nerves of the trunk and limbs. The spinal part is concerned chiefly with reflex actions initiated by activations originating in end organs, which respond to stimuli actually impinging on them. These end organs receive all the stimuli starting from the organs and tissues themselves, and also those of common sensation, including touch, pain, heat and cold and the like. Such reflex responses are direct single reactions to stimuli of a simple nature, and incapable of variation outside their special inherent character. That is to say, the reflex response, if not interfered with by disease processes, is always the same to a given stimulus. Therefore it is entirely predictable, and in itself cannot be altered by the individual, except in the case of those reflexes which have secondarily become subject to cortical control. Given the stimulus, the reaction is certain, but when over, that cycle of activity is finished, and only in exceptional circumstances leads on to a further cycle of activity. Though the response may involve several muscles and muscular groups it never results in complex behaviour. The brain proper, which is of later evolutionary development than either the spinal part or the vegetative system, and consists of all structures above the brain-stem, is, as Sherrington[1] has demonstrated, built up round the distance receptors. That is to say, it is concerned with the reception and elaboration of messages, coming from those end organs which receive stimuli from a distance, more particularly with the organs of sight and hearing. The end organs concerned with these senses are activated by "waves," which emanate from objects not in contact with the sense organs themselves. In addition to this, the functions of the brain are concerned with all the higher processes of thought, feeling and action. The brain may be divided into two essential parts, the subcortical region and the cortex. The subcortical part is concerned with the more complex reflexes, and perhaps with the simpler instincts. That is to say, the reaction may result in very complicated behaviour, and there may be some variation in the possible reaction, but this is very strictly limited. Consequently the reactions are fairly predictable, and are not in their natural state under the control of the individual. Such reactions may lead to a series of cycles of behaviour which may be hard to discriminate, but when once started, such an action, under its natural conditions, and when not controlled by the higher functions of the cortex, is carried out to the full with constant and invarying intensity. In other words, the function of the subcortical region obeys the "all-or-none" principle. The cortex, on the other hand, is concerned with what is usually known as voluntary action, and also with the association, correlation and integration of all sorts of messages from all sorts of end organs, so as to make possible the higher grades of mental process, which have to be considered later.

The essential element of the nervous system is the neurone or complete nerve cell. These cells vary in their characters in different parts, but all have the same structural plan. Together with special supporting cells—the neuroglia, which act as scaffolding—they constitute the whole mass of the central nervous system. The neurone consists of three parts, the receiving part or the dendrite, the central part or cell body, which is essential to the life and nourishment of the rest of the neurone, and the transmitting part or neuraxon. The dendrite is, as a rule, a much branched structure which enables the neurone potentially to receive messages from very numerous other neurones. The axon is, as a rule, less freely provided with branches; but in many cases, collaterals exist, whereby the messages may be side-tracked along paths other than that served by the main axis cylinder. In some cells, especially the association cells, within the central nervous system, the dendrite and axon are short, but in the case of the sensory cells and motor cells, serving the extremities of the limbs, these may be very long. The peripheral nerves proceed to all parts of the body, and are bundles of dendrites of afferent cells, and axons of efferent cells, belonging to the central and vegetative nervous systems. In addition to the strictly afferent and efferent cells of the nervous system, there are very numerous association cells within the central nervous system, whose function is to establish communications between the cells of different groups. Each nerve cell is a unity and is not structurally connected with its neighbours, though functionally no one neurone is independent of the rest. The point of contact is called a synapse, and there is much evidence to show that the synapses vary in the readiness with which they permit the transmission of activation. There is always more delay at this point than anywhere else in the course of the nervous path and under certain conditions, which are only dimly understood, the delay may be extended or diminished. When there is abnormal delay, or where the activation cannot pass over the synaptic junction, inhibition is said to occur. When there is abnormal hastening of transmission of the impulse, facilitation is said to occur. Inhibition and facilitation may be due to modifications induced in the pattern by the nervous activation itself, or more likely by modification of the fluid in which the synapses are constantly bathed. The constitution of this fluid is constantly altered, in relation to the altering constitution of the blood, depending on the activity, or otherwise, of the various organs of the body, and especially of the endocrine glands. It is probable, that when a synapse is reached in the course of activation, biochemical changes ensue which set up renewed activity in the next neurone. These biochemical changes naturally vary with the medium in which they take place. The exact nature of the activation of a neurone is still in doubt, but it may be observed as a change in electrical potential, "a wave of negativity," passing through the nerve cell and its processes. Although all the nerve cells which are going to function throughout the life of any individual, are present at birth, any given nerve cell cannot function unless and until its processes are provided with an insulating covering called the medullary sheath. Those neurones which are more recent developments in the course of evolution acquire this medullary sheath late in development. For example, the pyramidal motor system, which subserves the highest type of muscular movement, does not function for some time after birth in the human infant. This is because, the fibres of this system have not yet acquired their medullary sheath. Nor is the child capable of the highly specialized discriminated movements which depend on this system, until such time as the medullary sheaths are complete. The various neurones, although structurally independent, are not functionally independent; and it is found that even at birth, certain groups are so inherently constituted that the passage of activation across their synapses is facilitated. Such a group has been termed by Semon[2] an engram, which corresponds to the "schema" of English writers. After birth these engrams are modified and amplified, as the infant finds touch with, and is influenced by his environment. This occurs in such a way that inhibitions may arise within the inherited engram, so as to restrict activity in certain directions, or new facilitations may be produced so that the engram may join up with others, forming groups of great complexity. On the constitution of these engrams depends the behaviour of the individual. The new grouping may be temporary, or of a more or less permanent nature. In the latter case, well established habits of behaviour are formed which are difficult to alter whatever the circumstances. The new grouping depends on what is termed conditioning.

Reference has already been made to this process at the reflex level; let us take an example at a higher level. Certain of the inherited engrams subserve the reactions which McDougall[3] calls "instincts," but which we prefer to term emotional dispositions. Let us take two, the sexual and the fear-flight dispositions. Suppose a small girl has her sex impulse activated for the first time, by the assault of a tramp, in circumstances which produce extreme fear. The two engrams may be conditioned in such a way, that in future, sex can never be aroused without fear following in its train. If σ represents the sex stimulus, and S sex activity, and ϕ represents fear stimulus, and F fear-flight activity, normally σ results in (=) S and $\phi = F$ quite independently of each other but in the case cited, on one occasion σ and ϕ occurred together. Therefore $(\sigma\ \phi) = (S\ F)$ or sex activity may become inhibited altogether, and it may so develop that $\sigma = F$. This process is by no means uncommon, as has been shown by many psychopathological studies.

The simplest form of engram is the reflex, consisting of a motor response to a sensory stimulus, as has been described in the last chapter. Such reflexes may subserve, and their demonstration depend on the phenomenon of muscular tone, in virtue of which a muscle is held in readiness for action. Thus, if the tendon of the extensor muscle of the knee is tapped, the muscle contracts. This comprises the familiar knee jerk. The importance of the maintenance of tone in this muscle is manifest when we consider that it is the main agency in holding the leg rigid so that the erect posture can be maintained. On the other hand, certain reflexes have a more definite end in view, as for example the immediate blinking of the eye when a foreign body comes in contact with the sensitive cornea. This reflex preserves the delicate surface of the eye from damage. Reflexes also exist in relation to the vegetative system, as for example the relaxation of the sphincter of the bladder when the internal pressure in the organ has reached a certain degree. The fact that we have acquired a certain amount of control over this reflex is a secondary matter and has nothing really to do with the reflex, inasmuch as in certain spinal lesions, as a result of which all voluntary control is lost, the condition of automatic bladder is established, in which the bladder empties only when pressure has increased to a definite constant point, and always responds to this particular stimulus. Other reflexes have to do both with the spinal system and the vegetative system, and so reach a considerable degree of complexity, but it is characteristic of all reflexes that they do not enjoy a sufficiently complicated relatedness to involve consciousness, which is equivalent to saying in neurological terms that they are not represented on the cortex of the brain.

Mention has been made before of the Mass reflex which has been suppressed in man and is only demonstrated when the lower part of the spinal cord is freed from the suppressing effect of the higher centres. This reflex consists of a somewhat complicated response to any noxious stimulus of the lower limb. The leg is drawn up, away from the stimulus, sweating of the part occurs and the bladder is emptied. It will be seen at once, that in this case a somewhat complicated engram involving both vegetative and central nervous system neurones is concerned, but the engram, as such, is never active in a normal healthy man. It probably represents a low grade form of motor activity which was appropriate to some far distant ancestor which lived in water, but has become quite inappropriate to the human being. Yet the engram is still in being, and is able to manifest itself as a unity under very special circumstances. This retention of engraphic arrangement, while being totally suppressed because of its failure of adaptation to the requirements of the organism, is of great importance for psychology, as will be seen later, and its demonstration in the field of neurology gives important corroboration to what must otherwise have been somewhat speculative psychological theories. Consideration of such a reflex leads us to a principle in the working of the nervous system which is of importance, namely the principle of control, and the release phenomenon resulting from loss of control. This depends on the intervening neurones, at a higher level in the evolutionary hierarchy, between the afferent and efferent cells. In the lowest types of nervous system there is no such intervention, and consequently the response must always be "specific." That is to say, there can be no variation from a definite movement following a definite stimulus. Such stereotyped response is only possible when the nervous system and the requirements of the animal are of extreme simplicity. Very soon in the progress of evolution, the number of stimuli coming from within and without the animal become so numerous that a set of stereotyped movements of one muscle group for each stimulus would lead to inextricable confusion. Hence, the actions of the stimuli must be so arranged that several can be grouped together to activate a common motor path, and so produce an organized series of movements. In the lower animal, such as the earth worm, and primarily in the human embryo, the nervous system is segmentally arranged, so that a segmental stimulus normally evokes a corresponding movement in the same segment. Thus, Stimulus S induces an activation, which passes by afferent neurone A, through intermediate neurone I, to efferent neurone E, and so results in contraction of muscle M. But the activation may also spread along path I′, into the next segment, so that the muscle of this segment M′ is also activated. Again the activation may pass altogether from segment I, to segment II, so that M, the muscle of segment I, remains quiescent, while M′, that of segment II, contracts. This process may continue right up to the head end of the worm, until the neurones in the principal ganglion are activated. These have a controlling action on all the other neurones, in virtue of their organization and response to stimuli spreading from other neurones. As a result of this organization, the worm can move as a whole, the muscles of certain segments relaxing while others contract, so that the whole body wriggles along the ground; or, all the longitudinal muscles contract at once, so that the body is shot back into its hole on the approach of danger. These movements do not involve any consciousness or awareness, though, as is shown in the second chapter, they may be said to have their mental correlates. They are complicated patterns of response to certain more or less complicated patterns of stimuli. This process of side-tracking activation from one segment to the next involves the establishment of secondary arcs on the primary reflex arcs, such as have already been described, and the intervention of more neurones. As these processes become more complicated a whole series of arcs may thus be superimposed one on the other.

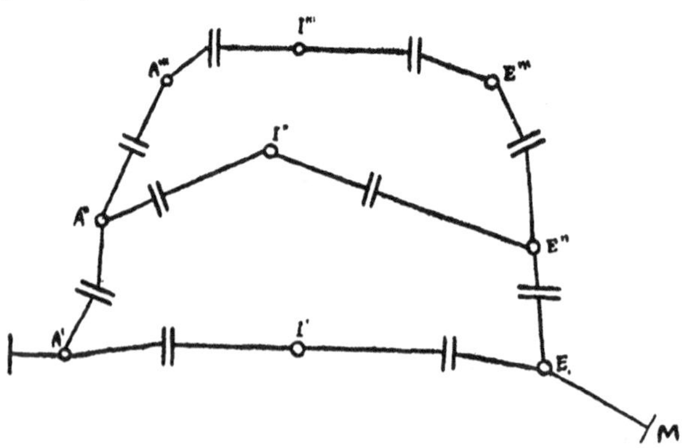

SUPERPOSITION OF ARCS
A=afferent neurone, I=intermediate neurone
E=efferent neurone, M=muscle

The passage of the activation through these higher series of arcs induces certain modifications. Firstly, there is delay in the response. This may be due to the necessity of passing a greater number of synapses, at which, as experiment has shown, definite delay does occur. Secondly, diminution in intensity of the response, since direct reflex response is always more violent than controlled response. This is true at all levels. For instance, the movements of the epileptic fit are movements in response to stimuli under conditions in which the control of the higher cortical levels is absent. Such movements are more violent, though less efficient than voluntary movements. The diminution of intensity of the response may also be due to passage through a greater number of synapses, if we compare the latter to a series of resistance boxes in an electric circuit. Thirdly, the intervention of higher arcs involves control and modification of response, owing to the possibility of "choice" of more numerous motor paths, which can act together or antagonistically or in series. This "choice" is not free but inherent in the engraphic arrangement of the neurones, either in accordance with original inherent dispositions, or as these are modified by contact with the environment. This brings us to discussion of a principle which illustrates the integrative and controlling function of higher levels. This principle is known as the law of reciprocal innervation of antagonistic action. We have to note that no action in the properly organized healthy individual is merely negative. Take for example a simple movement, such as extension of the wrist. At rest, the muscles supporting the wrist are not in a state of simple relaxation. On the contrary, they are maintained in a condition of static contraction, termed tone, whereby the wrist is held slightly extended and the fingers semiflexed. If the wrist is to be extended, not only are the extensor muscles contracted, but there is a definite inhibition of tone or relaxation in the flexors. This antagonistic action is well seen in the vegetative nervous system, in which the two divisions, the autonomic and sympathetic, are in every case reciprocal and antagonistic, the sympathetic accelerating the heart, while the autonomic slows it, the sympathetic dilating the bronchial tubes, while the autonomic contracts them, and so on. It is by this reciprocal action that such complicated mechanisms are involved, as that concerned with emptying the bladder. In this process while the muscles of the wall of the bladder contract, the sphincter, or closing muscle at the exit of the organ relaxes. It should be noticed, that efficient action is only possible when these antagonistic activities are properly integrated and balanced and this integration is one of the functions of the higher centres, especially of the cortex of the brain. This process of reciprocal action is of importance from the psychical aspect at higher levels, as will be seen when we come to consider such phenomena as the ambivalence of emotion. It is clear, that with the development of function of these higher levels, the original engrams are considerably changed in structure. How engrams which are inherently laid down at birth are modified is still obscure, but this modification unquestionably involves facilitation and inhibition. The innervation of vegetative neurones, and their resultant changes in the organs of the body, have some influence in inducing these phenomena. If these neurones are activated in certain ways, tension of certain of the involuntary muscles is induced. This, along with certain states of secretion in the glands and postural tone in voluntary muscles, may be said to make up a pattern of activation. Such patterns of action, with the accompanying efferent activities, vary enormously in accordance with the constituents involved, but all have a mental correlate. As part of this mental correlate there may be recognized degrees of feeling, or "affect." In the case of certain patterns of activation this feeling is one of ease or "pleasure," while in the case of others the feeling is of distress or "unpleasure". These affects, depending as they do on vegetative activity, determine to a large extent the permanence or impermanence of the engraphic arrangement of the neurones. Pleasure tends to facilitate their establishment, unpleasure tends to inhibit them. This process may be brought about indirectly by the intervention of modifications in the endocrine secretion. Further, if in the organization of the more complex engrams the addition of a given engram involves pleasure, it will tend to be amalgamated with the original, while if it tends to induce unpleasure it will tend to be divorced from the original. To understand pleasant or unpleasant affect, the quality of sensation, which also has an influence on the organization of engrams, must be considered. Sensations may be pleasant or unpleasant, and this quality depends on their intensity, the dividing line between the two varying with the sensation. For example, sweetness is pleasant up to a certain point, but after a certain intensity has been reached it becomes unpleasant. Similarly, with various other sensations, many of which are pleasant up to a very considerable degree of intensity. In the case of pain, on the other hand, the vast majority of the range of this sensation is unpleasant. However, very slight degrees of pain, such as that induced by the friction of the scalp with a hard brush, are pleasant. The distinction between pleasure affect and pleasurable sensation is sometimes made, and merits discussion. The former is usually described as dependent on the condition of relaxation, consequent on successful conation, while unpleasure is dependent on the condition of tension, or thwarted conation. This especially applies to instinctive reaction. Thus, the cat who has caught, killed and eaten a sufficiency of mice, sinks into a state of relaxation and may presumably be said to experience pleasure, while the hungry cat, who is prowling round in a vain search for mice, is in a state of muscular tension, and may be said to experience unpleasure. Such states of pleasure and unpleasure would seem therefore to depend on relaxation and tension of both striped and unstriped muscle, but it must be remembered, that when a muscle is in a state of increased tonus or tension a message as to its state of tonus is conveyed to the central nervous system, and is presented to it in the form of a sensation. In the case of pleasure the sensation will be of minimal intensity, and in the case of unpleasure of increasing intensity. This factor of intensity of sensation would therefore seem to be the fundamental factor, in determining whether affect is pleasurable or unpleasurable. Most examples of pleasure, even in its purest form, are already somewhat complex. For example, the performance of the sexual act is often quoted as affording pleasure in its most crude form. But even in this, there are three distinct forms of pleasure; the relaxation consequent on successful conation, i.e. pleasurable sensation derived from the enteroceptors, the sense organs concerned with reception of stimuli from the body itself; a definite pleasurable sensation in the ordinary sense of the term, i.e. sensation derived from the proprioceptors, the sense organs concerned with reception of stimuli from the environment in contact with the body; also, as will be pointed out later, pleasurable prospective imagination is involved, which is a function of much higher levels than those with which we are concerned at present. It must be remembered also that an engram may be altered, not only by actions which directly induce pleasure or unpleasure, but by actions which may secondarily induce these states. This brings us to a condition of more complex relatedness which may involve discrimination and therefore conscious, as opposed to unconscious activity. This may best be illustrated by a somewhat indirect analogy in behaviour. Suppose primitive man having reached the stage of eating cooked meat, accidentally discovers that the addition of certain white crystals which we know as salt is pleasurable, this pleasure is induced by the pleasant sensory response to a moderate intensity of saltiness, and also by certain changes in the muscles and glands of his digestive system, through the response of vegetative neurones to the chemical stimulus of salt, with their resultant sensory impressions. Salt is now sought for and the new primary engram induced by the stimulus of salt and the secondary engrams necessary to obtain salt are added to the original engram on which the eating of meat depended. But suppose he comes upon another white powder, say Tartar Emetic, and thinking it is salt tries it with his meat; the vomiting which results induces an affect of decided unpleasure. This unpleasure is again due to a different pattern of muscular and glandular activity responding to the chemical stimulus of the emetic. The engram becomes much more complicated, achieves a new relatedness, whereby discrimination is possible, and that part which involves Tartar Emetic as a stimulus is inhibited, so that he carefully avoids again taking Tartar Emetic with his meat. This complication of engram and the power of discrimination depends on an increase in the detail of the stimulus pattern, whereby certain visual and gustatory factors present themselves as different, and split themselves into two patterns, the stimulus pattern of salt being followed by facilitation of the engram subserving ingestion, while the stimulus pattern of Tartar Emetic is followed by inhibition of that engram.

These more complicated engrams then, from the neurological standpoint, involve a series of arcs superimposed one on the other, each "higher" arc delaying, diminishing the intensity of, and organizing and correlating the activity of the lower arcs. The evolution of the nervous system takes place, along the lines of a series of additions of higher arcs, at the front, or cephalic end of the nervous system. These higher superimposed arcs at the cephalic end constitute the "brain" at the various stages of development, though as has been said above, the term brain proper cannot be applied, till there develops some arcs higher than the brain-stem, whose function is essentially of the same class as that of the spinal cord. In the animal kingdom this represents the advance attained by the fishes, in which the appearance of a forebrain, corresponding to the basal ganglia, and the rudiments of a cortex is manifest. In the mammals we find the "neo-pallium" or cerebral mantle appearing. In the anthropoid apes, this has assumed a considerable degree of complexity and has so developed that the cortex has bent back and covers the whole of the rest of the brain. In man, not only is the size and complexity of the cortex increased, but two extra layers of cells are added. This means that the number of neurones, and consequently the potentiality for increased variation and complexity of action, is enhanced. It is calculated that in man there are nearly ten thousand millions of neurones, and if this figure is considered from the standpoint of potentially different combinations in engrams, the powers of adaptation in man's behaviour is explicable. It must be remembered that the inclusion of any given neurone in one engram does not preclude the inclusion in any number of others. Take as analogy a complex network of railways all over England. Any given stretch of line, say in Leicestershire, may be traversed by trains going from London to Carlisle, or from Cromer to Birmingham, or from Manchester to Bedford, or from Lincoln to Bristol, and so on, but yet there are perfectly definite routes laid down from London to Carlisle, etc. Such routes correspond to the engrams and the individual stretches of line to neurones.

A brief survey of the arrangement of arcs subserving the functions of motion, sensation and feeling will illustrate the sort of way in which the system functions.

In the case of motility, the primary path is the peripheral arc which is concerned with the maintenance of muscular tone in man, and is represented in the evolutionary scale by the segmental reflex of the earth-worm. If this reflex is interfered with, at any segmental level on the efferent side, the corresponding muscles lose their tone completely. If the afferent side is affected, then sensation in a corresponding area is lost, and the muscles partially lose their tone. This reflex is doubtless capable of integration up to a certain complexity, without the superposition of definite arcs, in some such manner as is represented by the mass reflex in man, already referred to. The next recognizable superimposed structure is the spinal arc, which reaches the brain-stem at the level of the upper part of the medulla, and establishes connexion with the cerebellum, a special structure which is chiefly associated with the functions of posture and balance. This spinal arc is, in man, associated with the maintenance of tone in the flexor muscles, which are concerned with the withdrawal of a limb from danger. In lower animals, however, this arc is concerned with the tone in the extensor muscles, whose function is to maintain the body raised from the ground, against the action of gravity. In the evolutionary scale, the establishment of this arc is probably related to the development of specialized limbs. The third arc is termed the prespinal arc, and establishes connexions at the level of the basal ganglia. In man this arc is concerned with posture and tone in the extensor muscles of the lower limbs, and the flexor muscles of the upper limb. Acting alone it allows certain movements of the limb as a whole, but the finer discriminated movements are impossible. In animals the reflex is concerned with the tone of the extensor muscles in all four limbs, and in the maintenance of posture against gravity, having an action similar to, but more efficient than that of the spinal arc. The reason of the difference between man and animals of function of this arc in respect of the arms is that the ancestors of man, in the direct line, had early depended on their fore-limbs for grasping and embracing movements. This development was in accordance with their arboreal habit, in contradistinction to the terrestrial habit of other animals, which requires that all four limbs should be used for locomotion. In the evolutionary scale this arc was efficient for those animals who only required that their limbs should move as a whole, as for instance the fin of a fish. The fourth and last definitely motor arc establishes connexions at the level of the cortex, in that part which is termed the Rolandic or motor area. This arc allows for fine discriminated movements, varying from the ordinary muscular movements involved in walking, to the fine discriminated "touch" of the expert pianist or violinist. The disturbance of any of the higher arcs releases the function of those lower in the scale, and it is largely as a result of the study of pathological cases that we have attained our knowledge of those lower arcs.

On the sensory side, in dealing with the proprioceptive system, we may follow up the same series of arcs and gain further knowledge by a study of sensory disturbances: (1) the peripheral arc, in which the cell bodies are situated in the posterior ganglia, just outside the spinal cord, and whose destruction involves complete loss of sensation: (2) the spinal arc, in which the cell bodies are found in the lower part of the brain-stem: (3) the prespinal arc, with cell bodies in the basal ganglia, and (4) the cortical arc, with cell bodies in the "sensory" cortex, situated just behind the motor cortex. It is interesting that the functions of the last two arcs involve a certain degree of awareness or consciousness, and that the basal ganglia and prespinal arc involve integration with impulses, travelling through the vegetative system from the enteroceptors. The series of arcs involved in this latter system is somewhat different; for the first arc involves cell bodies collected in ganglia, out among the viscera. The next arc has its cell bodies in the ganglia which form a chain on either side of the spinal column, and after a probable relay in the brain-stem, the final definite arc belonging to this system has its cell stations in the basal ganglia. Here then, these various types of sensation are correlated, and every sensation is accompanied with a greater or less degree of pleasure or unpleasure, as has been described above. Head[4] has shown that those sensations, whose perception involves much affect but little discrimination, are represented chiefly at the level of the basal ganglia. Thus pain is not seriously affected by the severance of connexions with the sensory cortex so long as the arc involving the optic thalamus is intact. On the other hand, those sensations whose perception depends chiefly on discrimination require representation on the cortex; and if this is interrupted, they are almost entirely lost. A good example of such a sensation is the sense of posture, for the position of a limb in space does not involve any particular feeling, apart from pressures and tension on painful spots, which are concerned with another sensation altogether.

It has been said that the basal ganglia represent the final cell station of the vegetative system. This is in a sense true, but none the less, the impulses which travel from the enteroceptors by this route are integrated with others to activate engrams whose mental correlates are emotions and sentiments, and these involve cortical representation. Apart from this however, the cortex does seem to have a controlling influence on the affective activities. Wilson [5] has shown that in lesions which interrupt cortico-thamalic connexions, the patient may have uncontrollable fits of involuntary laughing and crying, quite out of proportion to the stimulus, and unaccompanied by a corresponding conscious feeling of joy or grief. This illustrates an important principle, that activity at the level of the basal ganglia tends to be of the "all-or-none" variety; that is to say, if action of any sort results, it will be carried out with the maximum intensity of which the animal is capable. The final integration of activity of all varieties depends on the presence of the great association areas, which are the special feature in the development of man's brain, as compared with those of animals. The most important of these are the frontal lobes, and it is in these that the difference may be specially noted between the highly civilized man and the primitive savage. Little is known as to their exact function, but Bianchi [6] has performed some interesting and important experiments with monkeys. His findings in respect of the emotions may be taken as illustrative of the way in which these higher structures function. He found that those monkeys who were deprived of their frontal lobes retained their appetites, such as hunger, sex and panic fear, but that all the higher emotions and sentiments were lost. This was specially the case with all those emotional reactions, involving sociability and interaction with others of their kind.

We must conclude, therefore, that on the highest level of superimposed arcs depend all the complicated reactions of man, which are the special domain of psychology. It will be our duty to study these reactions, but we shall do so from the mental aspect, always assuming each reaction to have a physical correlate, depending on an engram, whose exact delimination cannot be determined, but whose nature and structure can be inferred from its analogy with those known to subserve activities at lower levels.

CHAPTER V

THE TEMPERAMENTAL FACTOR IN PERSONALITY

To the older writers, the various types of personality were distinguished according to the dominant "humour" of the body, and mankind was divided into four groups, corresponding to the four humours recognized by them. The sanguine person, in whom the blood was the dominant humour, was supposed to be light, superficial and accommodating. The melancholic, in whom black bile, whatever that was, dominated, represented the deep, self-involved, slow moving person—the strong silent man. The choleric person, with yellow bile dominant, was passionate, strong, and possessed of an active imagination; while the phlegmatic type, dominated by the colourless thick phlegm was dull, cold and slow—the "bromide" of a recent phraseology.

Such a division involved no little psychological insight into the different sorts of men, but it was impossible to demonstrate any facts to support the inference that these types had anything to do with the special variations in the liquid constituents of the body. The study of temperament thereupon came to be rather neglected; and, although it was universally recognized that bodily states influenced mental attitudes, the how and the why remained unanswered. It is a matter of common observation, that a grain of calomel may change a man from a hopeless pessimist into an unbridled optimist, but this is due to the clearance of the system from toxins which are directly influencing neural processes. It is probable, however, that there is more than this removal of toxins, for the immediate relief of mental strain which is sometimes experienced on movement of the bowels cannot be the result of depleting the circulation of toxins, a process which must involve more time. Whether we have any right to postulate any definite reflex action is doubtful, and this result may simply be due to suggestion. So, with the dysfunctioning of other organs, the toxins thus produced or retained within the body interfere with the general cœnesthesia or sense of well-being. This term cœnesthesia is used to describe a complicated sensory pattern from the enteroceptors, which considerably modifies the affective reaction to other stimuli. In the majority of cases, the influences of these poisons are temporary and pass away with their removal, but if the dysfunction continues, then there may be a permanent alteration in the personality. Such are familiar in the pessimistic, irritable chronic dyspeptic, the sufferer from chronic renal disease with his inconsequence, moodiness and depression, and so on. Such cases are directly comparable to those influenced by poisons introduced from without. Alcohol, morphine, cocaine and other drugs produce a transitory change in the reaction to the environment, if taken intermittently, but the whole character of the individual is altered if the ingestion becomes constant, and the subject is permanently under the influence of the poison. Such temperamental factors, then, belong to the realm of pathology and toxicology, and cannot be usefully discussed further here. However, a new interest has been introduced into the study of temperament by the increased knowledge of the action of the endocrine organs or ductless glands, which elaborate substances termed internal secretions or hormones. These organs are constantly present, and constantly pour their products into the blood stream, so as to affect neural function and consequently the manifestations of behaviour. Therefore, although a certain amount of excursion into the province of pathology is necessary to elucidate their action, it seems legitimate to study their influence on personality in greater detail. This is specially the case inasmuch as they influence growth, and as will be seen in later chapters, the departure of personality from the normal largely depends on abnormalities of growth, whether bodily or mental.

It is one of the fundamental characters of living protoplasm that it elaborates complex chemical compounds with a more or less specific action. On such substances depend the tropisms of unicellular organisms, the function of approach to food particles, and the retreat from noxious substances. Similarly, nervous action and transmission depend on biochemical substances elaborated within the cell, and at the synapses, which act locally at the point of liberation. The endocrine organs are specialized in this function and elaborate various substances, the so-called hormones, with definite specific actions, which act at a distance and influence the whole body. All these organs are well supplied with blood vessels and their products are absorbed into, and circulated in the blood stream, so that they are conveyed to all parts of the organism. It is arguable that all the organs of the body elaborate hormones, and the enthusiastic specialists in the subject claim that they can differentiate the functions of the hormones derived from the intestines, liver and so on. No doubt, when more fully understood, these hormones will be found to influence personality in definite specific ways, and their exact contribution to temperament will be elucidated. At present, however, their known action is purely physiological, and their psychological influence is undetermined or completely obscure. No purpose is to be gained, therefore, by discussing them, and it will be found more profitable to confine our attention to those whose action has been determined, both in the physiological and psychological fields, or in whose case the physiological effect is so far reaching that secondary psychical effects ensue.

It is one of the misfortunes of modern psychology, that the study of the action of the endocrine organs is one of such great complexity and difficulty. Everyone is agreed that these structures are of great importance in the regulation of both the bodily and mental activity of the individual, but, in spite of a very large literature which has grown up, exact knowledge in this sphere is still very restricted. Certain works which have been published in late years purport to give a clear picture of the mental and bodily alteration dependent on the excess or diminution of the secretory activity of the various glands; but many of the statements, especially in relation to mental factors, are of the nature of a priori probabilities, rather than of empirically proved facts and are consequently of very limited value. The difficulties which beset the path of investigators in this field are largely due to the fact that the system of endocrines work as a whole, so that, if one drops out, certain phenomena are met with which may be the effects of deficiency of the given secretion, or of the compensatory over-activity of others. Hence the exact function of one gland, or of a pair of glands, is hard to determine. Moreover, two given glands may act in co-operation in one respect, but in opposition in another. For example, the thyroid and the pituitary are both katabolic in function, that is, they convert potential energy into actual energy, and sugar from the blood will be mobilized for immediate use as fuel, if they are stimulated to activity. But the mental effects produced by overactivity of the thyroid are quite different from those consequent upon hyperpituitarism. In the former, the energy is dissipated in fretful irritable emotionalism, while in the latter, it may be used to foster a pushful ambitious efficiency. As Leonard Williams[1] has shown, the typical energetic American has the features of a very mild case of Acromegaly, a disease depending on the over-activity of the pituitary. For the purposes of this study, it may be best to try to indicate how the different glands influence the personality at various stages of growth.

Before and immediately after birth, metabolism and growth are said to be governed by the activity of the thymus gland, situated in the upper part of the chest, which normally ceases to function about the period of puberty, though some observers consider that thymic tissue persists to an advanced age. In man, this gland is developed from the third visceral pouch, an outgrowth from the alimentary tract, occurring at the time when the fœtus is passing through what may be described as the fish stage, since these outgrowths persist in the fish as the respiratory organs or gills. In man this pouch later takes on a lymphoid structure. The old idea, that this gland underwent involution about the second year of life, is not borne out by later investigation, and recent research shows that the activity and size of this organ has a certain direct relationship with that of the thyroid, so that it tends to undergo involution after thyroidectomy, and to increase in size in hyperthyroidic states. On the other hand, there is much evidence to show that the increase in growth and function of the reproductive organs hastens involution of the thymus, and any delay in development of the former leads to a persistence of the latter. Or, it may be that the reverse causal sequence is the true explanation, and one function of the thymus may be to act as a break on the development of the gonads. As may be gathered, exact knowledge of the function of this gland is not yet established, but deficiency of thymic secretion, due to extirpation in young mammals, causes a weakness of muscles, deficient calcifications of bones and general metabolic upset; that is to say, an interference with normal muscle and bone formation, which is the chief function of growth in the young child. On the other hand, overgrowth of the thymus frequently leads to sudden death from failure of the respiratory function, which may be the consequence of a resultant abnormal sensitivity to foreign proteins, or drugs. This is the condition known as status lymphaticus, which has been held to be responsible for many fatalities in children under anæsthetics.

The pineal body, a small structure embedded in the brain tissue, seems to have a similar inverse relationship to the sexual glands, as does the thymus, and destruction of the former by tumour leads to precocious sexual and mental development. It may therefore, also be responsible for the postponement of sexual function till puberty. It is to be noticed that only in the pineal type of sexual precocity does mental precocity occur as an accompanying phenomenon, and in view of this, it may be that its retarding influence extends to the more highly developed cortical cells, whose function is only required when the individual reaches a certain age. Little is known, however, as to the actual function of this gland.

Skeletal growth is considerably modified by the function of the pituitary gland, situated at the base of the skull. This consists of an anterior and intermediate portion, derived from an ectodermal invagination during early fœtal life, and a neuroglial posterior portion, derived from an outgrowth from the thalamencephalon, a part of the developing brain. Extracts from the posterior part, which contain a substance called pituitrin, exercise a marked tonic effect on plain muscle, especially in the circulatory system, and an increase in the activity of certain glands This, however, is a pharmacological action of transitory duration, and has no influence on the make-up of the personality. The presence of the anterior lobe seems to be essential to life, and diminution of its function delays growth of the skeleton and arrests sexual development. Over-function of the anterior lobe promotes tissue growth, especially in the skeleton, skin and subcutaneous tissue, and excites the development of secondary sexual characters. The hormone of the pituitary, therefore, promotes a continuance of growth and facilitates sexual development when the time comes for its full function. The disease acromegaly, which is characterized by marked overgrowth of the skeleton, is generally regarded as being due to hyperfunction of the anterior lobe. Insufficiency of the posterior lobe causes a slowing of metabolic processes. There is a high sugar tolerance, with the result that the storing up of carbohydrate induces adiposity. At the same time, the pulse and respiration rates are lower, and the blood pressure is diminished. These changes are specially marked in the hibernation of animals, and this phenomenon seems to depend on changes in the pituitary body, with diminished function of the posterior part. Insufficiency of pituitary substance, as a whole, causes the disease process associated with the name of Fröhlich. This is characterized by delay in skeletal development, great deposit of fat and persistent infantilism, i.e., the failure of development of primary and secondary sexual features. This is also accompanied by a childish mentality with a marked lack of initiative.

The records of the psychic effects of abnormalities of the pituitary gland are somewhat conflicting, and refer chiefly to the changes consequent on increased function of the anterior lobe. It would seem that mild increase in this is compatible with a good intellect, with an imaginative force which can be controlled and brought to the service of the subject's active brain; he is often musical, in short a practical visionary. However, even where skeletal development shows an overaction of the anterior lobe there may be a decided loss of control, and the patient is found to develop delinquent tendencies, such as lying and stealing. This may be due to the fact that there is a primary overgrowth of the gland, resulting in skeletal changes, followed by a secondary degeneration, resulting from the fact that the sella tursica—the depression in the skull, which contains the gland—is too small for the growing structure, and therefore induces a pressure fibrosis which destroys the active gland substance. There is a good deal of evidence to show that the anterior lobe is associated with masculinity and that the flat-chested, big-boned female, such as the French caricaturists used to portray as the typical English Miss, suffers from a too active anterior pituitary lobe. Such people are usually said to be unemotional, but this apparent want of emotion is due to an efficient control over emotional expression and impulsive actions. The fact that in many pituitary tumours there is often marked dullness and sleepiness, may depend on increased cranial pressure rather than on changes in the gland itself. Moreover, this sleepiness may be associated, to a certain extent, with the aggressiveness characteristic of normal hyperfunction of the gland. An example of this is afforded by the famous fat boy, who, when not asleep, strove to thrust himself into the lime-light by "making your flesh creep." It would seem therefore that cortical function, at its highest level, is dependent, at least to some extent, on a properly functioning pituitary gland.

The thyroid gland, situated in the neck, has a marked influence on metabolism all through life, and its function is perhaps better understood than that of the other endocrine glands, because its extract, given by the mouth, can be proved to have a definite metabolic effect, and because the diseases cretinism and myxœdema, on the one hand, are known with certainty to be due to deficiency of the thyroid secretion; while Graves' disease, on the other hand, is due to excess of this substance. Congenital absence of thyroid function gives rise to the type of maldevelopment, called cretinism, either of the myxœdematous or nervous type. In both types of this disease there is a marked inhibition of mental development, deaf-mutism being common. In the former type, the most characteristic features are the thick dry skin, stunted growth, and infantile characteristics; in the latter type there may also be certain physical neurological symptoms, such as spasticity, variations in posture, grimaces and other involuntary movements. As a whole the cretin is slowed down in growth, in mind and in bodily function, and if untreated, remains a dwarf and an idiot. Myxœdema is a disease due to deficient thyroid function, which supervenes in adult life. It is characterized by gradual swelling of the skin, which becomes dry and rough, sensitivity to cold, and an increasing languor and mental dullness. The mental changes may go on to hallucinations and melancholia, and the administration of thyroid will often benefit these latter conditions, even though they are not associated with definite physical signs of myxœdema. Here again there is a general slowing down of both bodily and mental function, and both these diseases may be improved, or even cured, by administration of thyroid substance.

Graves' disease, in which excessive function of the thyroid gland occurs, is characterized by an increase in the katabolic changes of the body, but the work done, as the result of this increased fuel destruction, all goes to waste for lack of organization. The signs associated with this disease are rapidity of heart action, acceleration of the respiration, excessive sweating, inco-ordinated function of the digestive system leading to nausea, vomiting and diarrhœa. The patient reacts excessively to all stimuli, and mentally and physically is incapable of co-ordinated effort. The result is excessive emotionalism, ready fatigue, and incapacity for sustained effort. This morbid syndrome is often capable of relief, or cure by extirpation of part of the enlarged gland. The relaticnship of thyroid activity to sexual life is still imperfectly understood, but it is certain that in the absence of thyroid secretion, sexual maturity is impossible, for untreated cretins remain infantile or sexually immature, and, in women at any rate, periods of sexual activity, puberty, pregnancy and menstruation, tend to increase thyroid activity. It is supposed, that the ovaries exert an inhibitory action on thyroid activity, and hyperthyroidism is often met with after extirpation of the former; but, although Graves' disease does sometimes develop after the menopause, it is much more common to find a deficiency of thyroid function at this time, the functions of both glands diminishing at this period of life. On the mental side, excessive emotional activity, especially if repressed, will result in an overaction of the sympathetic nervous system, and amongst other things produce hyperthyroidism. This pertains especially to the emotions of fear and anxiety, the reactions which are essentially concerned with increased sympathetic activity. In such cases a vicious circle is set up, for the increased thyroid secretion sensitizes and facilitates sympathetic reaction, so that the patient responds particularly readily to these emotions. The occurrence of moderate degrees of hyperthyroidism was remarkably common during the war, and represented the reaction of the thyroid system to fear and anxiety. We see then, that the thyroid secretion is necessary for the development and maintenance of nutritive, sexual, and mental function.

The parathyroids, separate glands in close anatomical association with the thyroid, have to do with the control of intestinal toxins, since their removal upsets the metabolic balance and allows the system to succumb to poisons. They are also associated with calcium metabolism and are essential to life. The existence of poisons circulating in the blood interferes materially with both bodily and mental function, and neither can be adequately maintained, unless the lime salts are in proper proportion. Apart from these factors however, the exact functions of these glands are so little known that they can hardly concern us here, in a study of Personality.

The adrenal bodies, situated in close contact with the kidneys, may next engage our attention. These consist of two parts, termed the cortex and the medulla. The former is mesoblastic in origin, while the latter consists of chromophil substance, a primitive embryological tissue, derived from the neural ectoderm, and concerned with the development of the sympathetic ganglia, as well as certain endocrine organs. By the study of Addison's disease, we may learn the effect of destruction of the adrenal glands. The symptoms of this morbid condition are extreme muscular weakness, low blood pressure, nausea and vomiting, along with increased pigmentation of the skin. In these cases the asthenia becomes so extreme that death eventually intervenes. This syndrome is found associated with disease of the adrenal bodies, usually tubercular in origin. Little is known with certainty as to the effects of increased activity of the glands, but high blood pressure and chronic interstitial nephritis, are often found to be accompanied by overgrowth of the adrenals. Whether the latter has any causal relationship, with the former, is not known. Recent experiments on animals, involving extirpation of the glands, give conflicting results, but it would seem that the cortex is the part which is essential to life. In transplantation experiments, most observers agree that the cortex survives, but that the medulla disappears. The latter contains an important substance known as adrenalin, whose physiological action closely resembles, if it is not identical with, that of the sympathetic nervous system, and is in most cases antagonistic to autonomic action. The chief features of its activity are constriction of the blood vessels with, acceleration of the heart, relaxation of the bronchioles, a liberation of sugar, and inhibition of vegetative or anabolic functions. All these effects prepare the animal for action, whether offensive or defensive, attack or flight, and there is no question, that the secretion of the adrenal medulla is increased in association with the arousing of the sthenic emotions, such as fear (panic) and anger. There is a certain amount of evidence to support the theory that this adrenalin is poured into the circulating blood, as the result of the reception of stimuli which arouse these emotional reactions, and reinforces and prolongs the nervous activity induced. For example, an asthmatic, in the course of an attack characterized, as all asthma is, by spasm of the bronchioles, was driving a motor car down a steep hill, when he suddenly found his brakes would not work. He experienced considerable fear, but having escaped destruction at the bottom of the hill, found that his asthma had disappeared. He usually experienced relief from an attack, by the administration of a dose of adrenalin, and there seems little doubt that the attack under discussion was cut short by a physiological dose of adrenalin, induced by the cognition of danger. The relationship of the medulla of the adrenal to the maintenance of blood pressure under ordinary circumstances is much more doubtful, and requires further investigation before a categorical answer can be given. On the whole, we may conclude that the action of adrenalin, like pituitrin, is pharmacological rather than that of a true internal secretion. The function of the cortex of these glands is still more doubtful, and various theories are held. It is tolerably certain that there is an intimate connexion between the sex characters and the adrenal cortex. Hypertrophy of this tissue is sometimes associated with precocious sexual development, and with the appearance of male characters in the female. Guthrie[2] described two types of cases of adrenal tumour with overgrowth of the cortex of the gland: (1) an obese type met with in both sexes with increased and precocious growth of pubic hair, but otherwise with little sexual precocity: and (2) the infant Hercules type, occurring only in males, who show true sexual precocity, but often mental defect. There is a good deal of evidence to support the theory that the adrenal cortex increases in size during periods of sexual activity and during pregnancy. Moreover, in structure this tissue closely resembles the interstitial cells of testis, ovary and corpus luteum. Feeding experiments in young animals point to the fact that the cortex exercises a stimulus to growth of the testis. The development of active suprarenal glands, within normal limits, will produce an aggressive virile type, similar to that depending on a good pituitary development, but overaction of these glands would seem to be associated with a dominance of fear and the occurrence of phobias, anxieties and the like. Under-development of the gland leads to weakness, submissiveness and feebleness of character. The adrenals maintain bodily and mental function in certain respects, and promote sexual development at the proper time.

The internal secretion of the reproductive organs are of very great importance in relation to personality. Removal of the testes in early life, or failure of development, leads to an arrest of the growth of the accessory sexual glands, viz., the prostate and the glands of Cowper; but more important than this, they lead to a failure in development of the secondary sexual characters, i.e., those physical and perhaps mental characteristics, which distinguish the man from the boy and the woman. Experiments on roosters have led Pezard[8] to conclude that these secondary sexual characters are maintained by a continual secretion from the interstitial cells of the testes, and that failure of the latter at any stage of development results in disappearance of these characters. These interstitial cells are distinct from the germ cells, are directly concerned with reproduction, and function as an endocrine organ. He also concludes that more internal secretion than is necessary is produced by the testicle to maintain these secondary sexual characters, since a small portion only of the testicle need be retained, to avoid their regression. Further, if secondary sexual characters are produced or maintained at all, they are maintained as a whole, and are not met with singly, or partially developed. Absence of testicular tissue leads to a persistence of infantile characteristics, and in no case to the development of female characters. Thus, in man, no hair develops on the face or on other parts of the body, the normal changes in the thorax and larynx do not occur, so that the voice remains high pitched, and the shape of the body remains that of the boy. It would seem, however, that the testicular internal secretion controls and inhibits the growth of bone and muscle in the body, so that early castration leads to gigantism. This is borne out by the observation that the Herculean man is often of low sexual potency. The presence of actively functioning testes seems also to control the accumulation of fat, which may account for the fact that eunuchs are almost invariably obese, and that on the whole, women are fatter than men.

Removal of the ovaries before puberty is a rare operation, and the records are inexact, but the result seems to be that not only do the usual secondary changes of skeleton, such as widening of the pelvis and characteristic fat distribution, not take place, but the woman takes on certain characters of the male, such as growth of hair on the body, low-pitched voice, etc. This would seem to indicate that the secondary sexual characters of the male are latent in the female, but are suppressed by the internal secretion of the ovary. It is to be noted that the converse is not the case, and that secondary female characters never develop in the male. The appearance of male characters after the destruction of the ovaries can be demonstrated in animals, as for instance, the growth of horns in female deer, and the development of anatomical and behaviouristic character in the hen, described by Crew[4] when the ovaries were destroyed by tubercular disease. Removal of ovaries after puberty results in an excitation of autonomic activity, in addition to the cessation of menstruation. This induces emotional disturbances, headache, fainting, intestinal derangements, and feelings of heat and cold.

Much has been written about the interrelationship of the individual ductless glands, and various syndromes involving two or three, have been evolved, whose intricacy is only equalled by the lack of evidence for their existence. These glands are derived from various sources, all three of the primitive layers of embryonic cells—ectoderm, mesoderm and endoderm—being represented. Hence there is no *prima facie* reason why they should work in such intimate relationship as many writers suggest, yet there can be no doubt that this specialized endocrine system does work as a whole, and interference with the function of one gland does show a repercussion on all the rest.

The thymus, thyroid and parathyroid are all derived from branchial clefts, and the glandular portion of the pituitary has a similar origin, though the former are derived from endodermal structure and the latter from ectodermal. The cortex of the adrenal is derived from mesodermal tissue, which is at least similar to that from which the gonads arise, while the medulla of the adrenals develops from the ectodermal chromophil tissue, from which the sympathetic ganglia also develop. Even in the case of those glands derived from the same embryonic cell layer, it by no means follows that there is a similarity in their physiological activities. There are however, certain indications which may be accepted with a due amount of reserve. The thyroid and adrenal medulla, both katabolic in their action, seem to work together, so that in hyperthyroidism more adrenalin is yielded to the blood. There is, however, no evidence to show that a diminution in thyroid activity is associated with alteration in adrenal function. When the thyroid is removed there is a considerable weight of evidence to show that the pituitary, also katabolic in its action, increases its functional activity; but it is doubtful if the secretion so induced is really a substitute for the deficient thyroid substance, for there is no increase of iodine, which is the chief constituent of thyroid secretion in the hypertrophied pituitary. The fact that the thyroid becomes enlarged at times of sexual activity, and that there is failure of sexual development in cretins, and frequently impotence in those suffering from myxœdema, points to the reciprocal stimulating influence of the thyroid and the reproductive organs. The effects of the increase or decrease of thyroid secretion, on other organs, is too doubtful to merit discussion here. With regard to the pituitary, absence or removal of this seems to result in increased activity of the thyroid, with a possibly indirect vicarious action. The pituitary seems to have a reciprocal effect with the sex glands, and also a compensatory action, and like the thyroid, it hypertrophies and increases its function at times of special sexual activity, while the same occurs if the gonads are removed. The adrenal cortex has a definitely stimulating effect on the sexual activity, and the function of the sex glands, especially in males; while the medulla would seem to have an antagonistic effect on the thymus and pancreas. Deficiency in growth of the sex glands seems to result in an overgrowth of the pituitary, perhaps by the absence of a normal inhibition with a consequent overgrowth of skeleton. The normal development of the sex organs at puberty checks the growth of the thymus, and seems to induce its retrogression, for castration results in a prolongation of thymic growth and activity.

The importance of abnormalities in sexual and bodily development is referred to in later chapters. It seems desirable therefore to draw attention to certain of these which are determined by temperamental factors.

Sexual precocity and its mental accompaniments

The appearance of puberty at abnormally early ages has been studied by many writers, and is apparently due to endocrine anomalies. The condition has been observed in connexion with tumours or overgrowth of the gonads, the pineal body, and the adrenal cortex. In the ovarian type there is an early development of primary and secondary sexual characters, menstruation often starting in the first few weeks of life. The mental condition does not keep pace with the physical development. On the contrary, there is usually a definite retardation in relation to the actual age. These children are generally small, with early closure of the epiphyseal junctions, at which the growth in the length of the bones take place. It is a common observation in normal women that those who menstruate early are usually short, and those in whom this function starts later in life are tall. This applies to races as well as individuals, as for instance in the Latin, as opposed to the Scandinavian women.

In the testicular type, there is similarly early development of primary and secondary sex characters, and often great muscular strength. The mental condition is retarded and the general control is poor, so that there is a tendency to delinquency, chiefly of the passionate and mischievous types. These children are also short, probably by reason of the inhibitory effect of gonadal secretion on pituitary activity, and consequently on the growth of the skeleton.

The pineal type occurs almost, but not quite exclusively in the male sex, and is the only form of sexual precocity associated with mental precocity. This latter is often astonishing, though if later the tumour of the pineal body produces intracranial pressure, various mental defects ensue. These children are reserved, shy and sensitive, and cry easily, and their general physical health is not robust.

The adrenal type tends towards masculine precocity. It is most commonly met with in the female, and leads to various male characteristics—development of hair on the face and body, enlargement of the clitoris and absence of menstruation. When it occurs in the male, there is marked precocity of primary and secondary sexual character, and a stature in excess of the normal. This latter feature distinguishes the adrenal type from the testicular cases. In mentality, all these cases are backward, and may be complete idiots. They tend to be aggressive and difficult.

Infantilism

By infantilism, is meant the retention of the characteristics of childhood up to an unduly advanced age, or a retardation of the rate of development. It is not necessarily associated with dwarfism, or arrest of mental development, but there is always delay or failure of sexual development. Various types are recognized; that most strikingly associated with endocrine defect, is the cretin, due to congenital lack of thyroid secretion, which has already been described. A second form of infantilism, is that associated with deficient pituitary secretion already referred to under the title of Fröhlich's syndrome. A third group is associated with intestinal disorders (Herter),[5] or deficiency of pancreatic secretion (Byrom Bramwell).[6] These cases show retardation of development in varying degrees, and all suffer from diarrhœa, with excess of fat in the stools. In Bramwell's case, the administration of pancreatic extract caused considerable improvement. Infantilism has also been observed in association with hypertrophic cirrhosis of the liver and chronic renal diseases, but the real causal factors in these conditions is obscure. Infantilism is met with in association with more general arrests and abnormalities of development, such as congenital heart disease, Mongolism and microcephaly, in which the condition under consideration is only a part of a general retardation. An interesting group are those described by Hastings Gilford.[7] They tend to appear in successive generations in a family, and form the greater number of what may be called the professional dwarfs. They perpetuate the facies of babyhood in adult life, and so tend to resemble each other closely. The head is relatively large, the face flat and wide, and the limbs short. Some eventually attain puberty, after long delay, but others remain infantile. There is no known etiological cause for this condition.

The relation of endocrine secretion to mental defect

It is quite certain that all cases of retarded mental development are not due to endocrine dysfunction, but there is an increasing body of evidence to show that there are types of mental defectives who show associated signs of endocrine defect. To attribute causative relationship to this endocrine defect is at present unjustified, for the latter may simply be part of a general arrest and abnormality of development. Mental defectives with endocrine abnormalities, can be classified into three groups: (1) The status lymphaticus group — slender loose-jointed children, with soft skin, poorly developed genitalia and a tendency to bed-wetting, and other infantile characteristics. The blood pressure is low, blood sugar below the normal and build under the average. These respond to a certain extent to endocrine therapy (small doses of thyroid and pituitary) gaining both in physical and mental development. (2) The hypothyroid group—short, stocky children with thick lips, flat noses and dry scaly skin. They are dull, lethargic and easily fatigued, listless, showing a low blood pressure and deficiency in blood sugar. So far as their personalities are concerned, no great change can be looked for from endocrine therapy (thyroid extract) if this is begun at all late in childhood, though a few improve quite definitely. If begun early in infancy, a cretinous baby may under favourable circumstances grow to be a normally intelligent child, fit to enter and hold his place in a public or secondary school. (3) The dyspituitary group; these are generally overweight, and big for their age, with irregularity of genital function, but normal blood pressure and blood sugar. These children are mostly irritable and unstable, with a tendency to sluggishness. Only rarely do they respond well to treatment by pituitary substance.

Potter, in his investigation at Letchworth village colony, found a moderate degree of improvement in many cases belonging to the type described above, while under endocrine treatment. His results seem to justify the conclusion not only that the endocrine function is an important contributory factor in determining arrested mental development, but also that in some cases, the lack of this can be, at least partially, remedied by artificial provision of the required glandular extract.

Dwarfs

Many authors divide dwarfs into those who are normal in proportion, and those who are disproportioned. In some cases the deficiency in stature is associated with infantilism, but not always so. In the first group of well-proportioned dwarfs, there are those who are described by von Hausemann[8] as "too small from the beginning" and those in whom growth is arrested at some period of development. These persons are normal in proportion, and resemble men and women seen from the large end of a telescope. They are not infantile as a rule, and may propagate their kind, but such anomalies as undescended testicle are not uncommon. Similarly, their mental capacity is good, and corresponds to their age and not to their size. The cause of the retardation of ossification, which is responsible for the condition is not understood.

Another type of symmetrical dwarf is that associated with injury, or deficiency of the pituitary. These have symmetrical skeletons, infantilism, and a normal mental equipment. They show a broad skull and a widely open jaw angle. The general resistance of these persons is fair, and though their bones are small, they are relatively strong. In contrast to this type, is that described by Sternberg[9] as hypoplastic dwarfism, in which there is a deficiency of all the ductless glands, as well as other organs, such as the brain. In these there is a symmetrical skeleton, infantilism, deficiency of mental power, and lowered general resistance of the body, coupled with feebleness of bones and muscles. The skull is not broad, as in the last type, since the brain is not fully developed, and so does not require the compensatory enlargement of the cranial vault. Dieterle[10] and others describe a dwarfism due to deficient thyroid secretion, differing from cretinism. Although there is a tendency for growth in length to be deficient, and growth in breadth to be normal, this is not always so. The probability is that some other factor besides deficiency in thyroid secretion is involved in these cases. Gigon[11] describes dwarfism due to failure of cerebral development. This may be symmetrical, or certain parts, such as the left arm, may be dwarfed with corresponding failure of development of the associated area of the cerebral cortex. These show marked mental deficiency and often other cerebral disturbances, such as epilepsy. Stier[18] maintains that in cases of partial dwarfism the deficient limbs are those in association with the "inferior hemisphere," i.e. the right hemisphere in right-handed persons, and the left in left-handed. Whether this failure in cerebral development is a primary variation, or secondary to endocrine defect, is uncertain. Dwarfism is also found in Mongolian idiots, a form of cerebral mal-development associated, at least in many cases, with congenital syphilis. Similarly in other forms of idiocy, growth and general development are definitely deficient.

The second group of deformed dwarfs, comprises the true cretin, and certain dwarfisms, due to definite diseases.

The cretin, as has been described above, is due to deficiency in thyroid secretion. The skin is thick, the tongue and lips enormous, the legs crooked, and the spine abnormally curved. These cases if untreated remain infantile, and hopelessly mentally deficient. The adequacy of normal nutrition plays an important part in the determination of dwarfism. For example, achondroplasia is a disease characterized by failure of growth in length of the long bones. The head and trunk are of normal size, but the limbs are stunted. Sexually they develop normally, and mentally are usually up to the average. The condition is supposed to be due to anomalies of nutrition in intra-uterine life.

Rickets, a disease of nutritive deficiency in childhood, so affects the growth of the bones, that deformity and dwarfism is a frequent result. In these cases sexual and mental development are usually normal.

Gigantism

Giants like dwarfs, may be divided into two groups—symmetrical giants and deformed giants. The former are normal in health and development, except for their unusual size.

In certain cases gigantism is associated with disturbances of the pineal gland; and in such cases, there may be both sexual and mental precocity, with no abnormality of proportion in the skeleton. Eunuchoid gigantism is associated with failure of development of the genital glands. Such persons show a poor mental equipment, and often certain skeletal anomalies, such as genu valgum and saddle nose. The commonest type of gigantism is associated with overgrowth of the pituitary gland, the so-called Acromegaly. If this occurs in youth, before the epiphyseal junctions are closed, a more or less well-proportioned gigantism results, but there is always a tendency to special growth of hands, feet and jaw. If the disease comes on in adult life, there is no increase in stature, but the latter enlargements only are met with. Such cases are, as a rule, definitely in bad health. The muscles are poor and flabby, the bones porous and often brittle, and the mentality low in most cases. The genitals are normal in size i.e., small in proportion to the size of the body, and their function is often, though not always, deficient. Deformities due to spinal curvatures are common, due chiefly to the weakness of muscles and supporting structures.

Gigon [11] maintains, that just as cerebral deficiency may lead to general or localized dwarfism, so cerebral hypertrophy may lead to general or localized gigantism.

These examples show the importance of temperament in general, and of the endocrine glands in particular, in influencing the equipment of the personality, both mentally and physically. Also it will be evident that our knowledge of the exact function of these organs is woefully deficient, and that if the future brings us a clear understanding of the interaction of the nervous system and the endocrine glands[13-14], many problems in the study of personality, and its multifarious reactions will be solved. For the present, however, it is not fruitful to pursue this subject further, and we must proceed to the study of higher mental integrations.

CHAPTER VI

THE INHERENT ORGANIZATION OF MENTAL FUNCTION

HAVING established the principle of temperamental influence, and having indicated how the different hormones reinforce and modify neural function, we must return once more to a consideration of the latter. It is however necessary to change our point of view, though, in passing from the consideration of bodily function to that of mental function we do not alter the subject of study, but only the aspect from which we study it. Heretofore we have been chiefly concerned with the more lowly organized patterns, whose physical aspect was presented for our study, but whose psychical aspect was of such a low order of organization that it failed to have significance. We might continue to attempt to follow the engraphic physical structure of the more complex mental patterns, together with the temperamental factors which influence their function, but this would lead us into such a complicated maze of neurones that our efforts would be fruitless; especially as the exact function of the higher cerebral realms, such as the frontal lobes, are still beyond our grasp. For this reason, it is more useful to concentrate on the psychical aspect, and transfer our attention from physiology to psychology. This is the more important, inasmuch as at these higher levels it is the psychological and not the physiological aspect which is significant; and in order to be intelligible, it is necessary to describe and examine behaviour according to psychological laws. In this sense it is legitimate to talk of an animal being guided by instinct, or by reason. This does not mean that we regard instinct or reason as having any force or influence of themselves. All that is implied is that the behaviour of the animal is a function of the activation of that engraphic pattern, which involves instinct or reason, and which is significant in virtue of that instinct or reason.

At these higher "mental" levels, the organization of the engram involves both central and visceral systems, on the afferent and efferent sides, and hence we can always recognize three phases in the processes under discussion. These are an afferent phase or cognition, involving the mental aspect of the reception of the incoming stimuli; a visceral phase or affect, involving pleasure or unpleasure; and an efferent phase or conation involving the mental aspect of the urge or "wish"* towards activity. These phases of cognition, affect, and conation are always present in every mental process, but may be differently stressed, and occur in different proportions.

As has been said already, the lower grades of mental activity are hard to describe because they are not open to clear introspection, not having achieved that organization which involves full consciousness. Moreover, in ordinary life they have, as a rule, been organized or fused into higher processes, so that they only appear in their primary form under exceptional circumstances. It will be remembered that in the discussion of the nervous system, it was pointed out that organization tended to be in the form of pairs of opposites, so far as the efferent or conative phase was concerned. This is specially the case in the vegetative system, where the sympathetic and the autonomic systems function antithetically, each producing the opposite effect to the other. Similarly in the projicient system, which has to do with the organization of voluntary muscular action, the muscles are arranged as agonists and antagonists, one group relaxing while the other contracts. It is not surprising therefore to find that, in the higher organizations, conation tends to appear as pairs of opposites. This is specially so in those patterns which subserve organic needs, and of which the visceral neurones form the most important constituent. The same is true of the affective dispositions, which at higher levels involve emotional life, since they also involve visceral activity which is most typically bipolar from the beginning. As has been pointed out, the transition from the reflex stage, in which an animal is little more than a plaything of circumstances, responding in a special way to any stimulus which impinges upon it, involves a new

* "Wish" is here used in the technical sense introduced by Freud, which, as Holt pointed out, was a real contribution to Psychology, as giving a name to the unit of conation.

emergence—viz., that of mind, and requires a new anatomical structure, that of brain, as opposed to the purely segmental nervous system. With this new structure and new function, two new factors are introduced, namely enjoyment * and initiation of effort. This enjoyment and this initiation of effort need not be conscious, but even at the level of appetite, we talk of feeling or of experiencing, technically enjoying, hunger. If we study the decerebrate dog, who has no brain and no mind, we find that if food is placed in his mouth, he eats it, but will go on eating without reference to the enjoyment of hunger. Further even if food is placed near him he will not take it. These new factors seem to depend on the more complex organization at this level, in accordance with the law of emergence.

The first processes which call for discussion, are the appetites of hunger and thirst. The stimulus pattern, from which the cognitive phase of these processes is derived, is received by the enteroceptors, the sense organs of the viscera, in the form of certain kinæsthetic sensory impulses from unstriped muscles, innervated by the vegetative nervous system. The affective phase is almost pure unpleasure, while these tensions are unrelieved, and pure pleasure when the appetite is satisfied, and tension is relaxed. The conative phase is the urge towards activity, which will satisfy the organic need of food and drink. This may result in the most complex behaviour in those animals who live in the medium where food has to be sought and won. Such complex behaviour however, is secondary, for the obtaining of satisfaction is a much more simple process when the animal lives in the all-pervasive medium of water, which was certainly the habitat of the earliest forms of life. In the majority of cases it meant that a volume of the surrounding medium was engulfed, and the fortuitous presence of organic material in it, satisfied the need.

The opposite to this hunger appetite is a process which requires mention at this level, and which may be described as the act of repulsion This has a definite cognitive phase, which is met with in the youngest infant, and depends on the reception of stimuli from visceral tensions of overstretched plain muscle fibre. It is difficult to give a name to this, but it is the experience involved when an overfull hollow

* Enjoyment is used in Alexander's sense as a technical expression for what might be expressed colloquially as experiencing.

viscus requires a discharge of its contents. It is the obverse of the appetite, since it is expulsive instead of appetitive. The affective phase is an especially differentiated state of unpleasure which, in the case of the stomach, is termed nausea, and the conative phase leads to contraction of the viscus, with correlated reflex closing of one opening and relaxation of another. For example, in the case of the stomach, the organ contracts, with the opening of the communication to the gullet, and the closing of the communication with the bowels as accompaniments.

The next process to consider is the sex appetite which is more complex, since it is a composite of appetitive and expulsive dispositions. It must be pointed out, that though sex appetite is regarded as pleasurable, it is only the consummation that is so. The preliminaries involve tension, and tension is always unpleasant. It is only when the conscious level is reached at which imagination begins, that the whole process is pleasant. As McDougall[1] has pointed out, imagination is typically anticipatory, and this is so in virtue of the engraphic patterns, already laid down. Thus, once the activation has started at the conscious level, "the end is in view," in virtue of the short cut process of thought and imagery, which will be discussed later. This anticipation involves such intense pleasure, that it quite outweighs the unpleasure of the preliminary tension. In the sex appetite, the appetitive and expulsive conations would seem at first sight to be differentiated in accordance with sex difference; the conation to fill a hollow viscus, being the female part, and to empty a hollow viscus, the seminal vesicles, the male part. However, as we shall have occasion to discuss more fully later, the sexes cannot be rigorously separated, either structurally or functionally, even on the physiological level of simple organization, still less on the psychological level of complex organization. So we must allow both in the male and female sex appetite, a bivalent rôle of appetition and expulsion, with an affect of unpleasure before consummation, which is overshadowed by the anticipatory pleasure at the conscious level.

The importance of these visceral tensions, based on the primary appetites as underlying factors in our behaviour, will be referred to later, when discussing Kempf's contribution to the study of personality.

At much the same level as these simple appetites, may be placed the processes of primitive fear, and primitive anger, whose conations of retreat and aggression are likewise a pair of opposites. These are not experienced by individuals under ordinary circumstances, being as a rule fused, to constitute higher level reactions. When they do appear, they have not such a high organization, either on the cognitive or conative sides, as have the usual expressions of the appetites already discussed. As organized and experienced in human consciousness, the three latter appetites are characterized by a knowledge of what is the matter. We know that we are hungry, thirsty or lustful, and as a sequence of the conation, we plan out discriminated behaviour to obtain food, drink or mate. Moreover, we are able to exercise control, so that these various activities may be modified to any extent, or inhibited altogether. This is only another way of saying that these appetites may be, and usually are, organized on the level of consciousness or cortical function. This is not the case however with the processes about to be discussed. Panic fear only occurs under overwhelming stimulus, which is strong enough to involve a dissociation, of personality; or in the course of neurotic illness, when dissociation, and abolition of full cortical function, are the chief characteristics of the pathological process; or again, in gross lesions of the cortex. For instance, Bianchi[2] describes this unreasoning fear as occurring characteristically in monkeys whose frontal lobes have been destroyed. This process of panic is characterized by a cognition of danger to the ego, but there is no knowledge of what this danger is, nor discrimination in time and space as to when and where the danger arises. The affect is intense unpleasure, with very marked increase of tension, and this is so organized with the efferent conative pattern that the resulting impulse is to escape anyhow, in any direction. This process, as seen in the neurotic, does not show the normal conation. The activation of the efferent neurones is inhibited, with the result that there is a short circuiting through the visceral neurones, with the most distressing and violent unpleasant affect.

Primitive anger is never exhibited under ordinary circumstances in human behaviour, but probably the condition not uncommon among certain primitive people, especially in the Malay Archipelago, known as running amuck, is a pathological unmasking of this process. In this case the cognitive process may be set off by almost any stimulus, whether actually thwarting or threatening the individual, or not. The affective unpleasure is so organized with the efferent conation, that the most violent aggression results, with every effort directed to destroy any object that comes in the path.

As integration and differentiation proceed, in the course of evolution, a disposition is laid down which McDougall[3] has referred to as primitive passive sympathy. This is present to a certain degree in all animals, and, as will be seen later, is integrated and differentiated to a remarkable extent as evolution proceeds. The cognitive phase is represented by the reception of afferent impulses, derived from stimuli arising from some other member of the animal kingdom, whether in the form of a cry or a movement. The affective and conative phases are considerably differentiated, as the tendency is for similar engrams to be activated in the recipient of the stimulus, as are being activated in the originator. Examples of this may be observed by watching the behaviour of other rabbits in a warren, who have seen the warning spectacle of the disappearing white tail of one of the tribe who has scented danger. Or again, of the wolf pack, hearing the hunting yelp of one member who has scented prey, and so on.

An obverse of the primitive passive sympathy may be postulated, in which the affect and conation are the direct opposite to that of the originator of the stimulus, but this is not readily observed, unless it be in the negativism of children and neurotics. In this state, the recipient feels and does exactly the opposite to the originator, but negativism is certainly a derivative, and not a direct manifestation of the obverse of primitive passive sympathy. In Chapter IX the phenomenon of the ambivalence of the emotions will be discussed. In this connexion, there seems a general tendency for affective dispositions to occur in pairs of opposites, which are readily translatable one from the other; therefore, at least on a priori grounds, it seems probable that there is such a primitive disposition, though not readily observable in ordinary behaviour. It may be noted that these last four dispositions are essentially built up round the organization of the distance receptors, and therefore necessarily involve the level of the brain proper, and a certain degree of cortical function.

Next in order of integration come those inherent engrams subserving patterns of behaviour, which McDougall[3] has termed instincts. It has been suggested that the term "emotional disposition" might be better, inasmuch as McDougall's instincts are rather more highly organized than are those dispositions in animals to which the term instinct was originally applied. Moreover the latter term was used to connote a disposition less easily modified by contact with the environment than are McDougall's primary units. This point however is of no very great importance, since too much stress cannot be laid on the fact that man's personality and behaviour depends on "instincts," strictly comparable to those of the animals, and not on some peculiar faculty of reason or free will. Whatever term we use, McDougall describes seven of these dispositions as primary. They are characterized by an organization of the three phases referred to above, on the cortical level. The cognitive phase, by means of which the subject is aware of the nature of the stimulus, is definite, and as a rule, the degree of the stimulus and its situation in time and space are distinguishable. The affective phase is characterized by an emotion,* that is to say pleasure or unpleasure, differentiated as to nature and degree, and organized with a conscious cognition, and a more or less controlled and discriminated conation. The conative phase is so organized, with the affective phase, that it results in a more or less specific pattern of behaviour, which is typically under conscious control. As has been said in Chapter IV, affective reactions have much to do with facilitation and inhibition, and so influence both the quality and quantity or force of conation; so that for this reason the emotions are often referred to as the springs of behaviour. Such characteristics show that these dispositions are organized on the level of full cortical function, that is to say, they are fully conscious.

It is not necessary to discuss these very fully here, since this has been done so admirably by McDougall himself, and by others who have followed him.[4] All that need be attempted is to indicate the organization of mental process in gradually increasing orders of complexity.

The disposition which McDougall describes as the instinct of flight is derived from primitive panic, by means of greater organization and discrimination. The cognitive phase, at this level, allows for a certain amount of dis-

* The term "emotion" is too loosely used in psychological literature. Here it is suggested that the word may connote affect organized on the cortical level, and integrated with conscious cognition and conation.

crimination, as to the nature and degree of the stimulus, and similarly, the affective phase allows of discrimination of degrees of fear experienced. So far as the conative phase is concerned, this is more or less specific in most animals, according to the species. Thus, the horse runs away, the rabbit runs and hides, the hare remains motionless, and only runs as a last resource. But as Rivers[6] has pointed out, this conation may be differentiated in man to a considerable extent. The resultant behaviour may be flight, or concealment, or a transformation to the conation belonging to another disposition, namely aggression. Again it may be transferred to a much higher level, and result in complex manipulative activity, or it may sink to a low pathological level, and appear as complete collapse. This means, that the conation is under the discriminative control of cortical function, except in the last case, and that in virtue of this higher and more complex organization, man is freer in his action than are the animals.

Similarly the disposition to aggression, in the presence of some thwarting of a conative effort or wish, is an organization of primitive anger, on a higher level, with greater specificity, differentiation and control, in all three phases.

Curiosity is an emotional disposition, which has been evolved from the appetites of hunger, and perhaps sex, when the rise in evolutionary differentiation necessitated the search for food, drink and a mate. The cognitive phase consists of the reception of stimuli from something strange. The affective phase, which McDougall calls wonder, leads to a conative phase, in which the strange object is approached. That this approach was originally for the purpose of satisfying the appetites may be inferred from watching a goat or a cow approach a red petticoat hung on a line. Curiosity is obviously aroused, and if the panic reaction is inhibited—for a strange object may activate this engram, as well as that subserving curiosity—she proceeds to chew it vigorously until such time as it is obvious that it is not satisfactory as a means of relieving hunger, when it is dropped and curiosity in respect of it ceases. Later, with further discrimination of all three phases, neither cognition or conation may have anything whatever to do with the primary appetites, the conation being conditioned to respond to some other stimulus and serve some other end, but such modifications are of course constant in evolutionary progress.

The disposition of repulsion, with its emotion of disgust, is clearly derived from the disposition of the overfull hollow viscus, in this case the stomach, to expel its contents. It must be realized however, that in the stomach the physical process of antiperistalsis, with its affective reaction of nausea, may be set up, not only by mechanical overfilling, but by the presence of irritant material in contact with the mucous membrane. Secondarily, in accordance with the law of the conditioned response, the same reaction may be experienced in relation to certain odours, often erroneously described as tastes, and even to sights and sounds. Hence the range of stimuli giving rise to the cognitive phase of this disposition is widened and differentiated to a considerable extent, while the conative phase is also more differentiated and controlled than in the primitive expulsive reaction described above, for disgust by no means necessarily involves vomiting, any more than fear necessarily involves flight.

The parental or protective disposition, is derived from primitive passive sympathy, organized with a reaction which was primitively at the reflex level, namely the suckling of the young. The excretion of milk, in response to sucking or pulling of the nipple, is a true reflex, and it is while this is in action that the parental instinct in its most simple form can be observed. It may be objected that many, if not most, of the examples of the parental disposition in operation, have nothing to do with the suckling of the young, but it is a well-established fact that, in the course of evolutionary progress, many reflex and analogous processes are diverted from their original end, both on the afferent and efferent side. It is important to realize that the suckling reflex, in common with the other excretory reflexes, is centrifugal in respect of the ego. Moreover the reflex of giving milk, started by the contact of the lips of the offspring with the nipple, is of a different category from others, inasmuch as it is essentially related to the behaviour of another individual. It is this which conditions and changes the affect, but specially the conation of passive sympathy, so that it emerges as something different and characteristic, as an altruistic impulse, according to the strict law of emergence. Another objection might be raised, that the parental disposition is just as characteristic of the male as it is of the female, and therefore cannot depend on the purely feminine activity of suckling. But in Chapter XI we shall have occasion to point out, how the sexes are much less differentiated, both physically and psychically, than is at first sight apparent, so that, an archaic reflex such as the one under review, may easily be manifest as a contribution to the emergence of a disposition in man, as well as in woman. Moreover every man has vestigial mammæ, which occasionally are able to function to a slight extent. From this it may be inferred, that there is at least a potential organization of an engram subserving their function. In support of this we may refer to the story quoted by Darwin, of the man whose wife was suddenly killed while nursing her child, and who was able to rear the infant, by the secretion of milk, induced by the continual stimulus to his own breasts. As organized in the parental disposition, the cognition is derived primarily from the movement, smell or cry of the offspring, but secondarily, from anything small and unprotected. We have no special word to describe this affect, but McDougall terms it tender emotion. The relation of this to sympathy is obvious, inasmuch as we tend to experience the same emotion as does the object of our tender feeling. The conation may be complex and varied, but its primitive form may be inferred from the mother clasping her child to her breast, or the tendency of the ignorant mother to give her baby the breast whenever it cries. At higher levels, the conation is directed to the protection and cherishing of the object which originates the cognition.

The dispositions of self-abasement and self-assertion are difficult to place. Many writers are agreed that they are much too complex to be classed as primary, though their successful analysis is by no means easy. Under the principle of emergence however, this may be attempted. In the composition of self-assertion, there is unquestionably aggression, and the conative behaviour of self-display is quite easily transformed into frank aggressive attack; yet it is aggression modified and conditioned in a remarkable way. The cognitive phase is derived from stimuli, arising from objects in the environment, weaker than the subject, especially from living organisms, who are exhibiting behaviour dependent on the opposite disposition, self-abasement. The affect and conation are the direct opposite of the latter, and in accordance with this it is suggested that, in this case, aggression is combined and conditioned by that disposition described above, as the obverse of primitive passive sympathy. Moreover, the appetites may have contributed to the organization of this disposition in its primitive form, for the conative behaviour, or self-display, early becomes an adjuvant to the obtaining of food and winning of a mate and as Darwin has shown, display soon becomes almost a secondary sexual character.

Self-abasement certainly involves panic and retreat, but this is modified and conditioned, just as aggression is modified, in self-assertion. Here the cognitive phase is derived from stimuli arising from something threatening in the environment, especially if it is exhibiting self-display, and the affect and conation is the direct opposite; so again, the obverse of passive sympathy is a factor in the emergence. In addition, just as the appetites may have had something to do with self-assertion, so the expulsive disposition may contribute to self-abasement. At any rate, the emptying of a hollow viscus is a frequent accompaniment of self-abasement, as can be seen by watching the behaviour of a puppy. It is conceivable that, as in self-assertion, when part of the conative effort is to achieve and receive something, the appetite impulse is dominant; so in self-abasement part of the conative impulse is to propitiate and give something, and hence the expulsive disposition may be dominant. Incidentally, certain of the Freudians maintain that the excretions are regarded as a propitiatory donation, but such contentions must be left *sub judice*. As further evidence that the disposition of self-assertion and self-abasement are highly organized, it may be pointed out that both tend to avoid expenditure of energy. An animal, by self-assertion, frequently achieves an end which would otherwise require great effort in the form of a fight against an enemy, or the pursuit of a mate. Similarly by self-abasement, he may achieve safety for himself, which would otherwise only be won by fighting or flight. Professor Janet[6] pointed out, that it was characteristic of behaviour at higher levels that there was a saving of actual energy, though there might be great potential energy involved in the process. The use of language exemplifies this, when we compare the energy expended in expressing our meaning by a word, or by pantomimic gestures; or again, as Varendonck[7] has shown, when we use selective memory, as opposed to reduplicative memory, in which every detail is recalled. Inasmuch then, as these dispositions save expenditure of energy, they represent behaviour at a high level, and the primary status claimed for them by McDougall should not be accepted too readily.

In addition to these seven "primary" dispositions, which have well-marked cognitive, affective and conative phases, McDougall recognizes several others. Suggestion, sympathy and imitation would seem to be organizations of the three phases of primitive passive sympathy, with a certain degree of self-abasement. Suggestion, which is the cognitive phase, is fully discussed in connexion with the neurotic personality. Active sympathy which is essentially affective, differs from passive sympathy in its more elaborate differentiation, and by its being under the discriminating control of cortical function. Imitation again, is the more controlled and differentiated conation, which is exactly comparable to the behaviour of the rabbit or wolf quoted above, who whole-heartedly copies the behaviour of the originator, in his flight from danger, or his pursuit of prey.

The gregarious instinct, which is only characteristic of certain animals including man, has, as its cognitive phase, a negative stimulus, in the shape of absence of others of the species, but this also involves a certain amount of cognition of danger. The affect is an organization of tensions, involving unpleasure, for which we have no name. The conative phase, in its original form, constituted an impulse to gain close physical contact with other members of the herd, as when a buffalo, which has been left behind, on regaining the herd worms his way into the very centre, as though he would apply every part of his body to the living flesh of his mates. This would appear to be an organization of panic flight, with primitive passive sympathy, in a new relatedness. This new emergent is of great importance in man, and has undergone modification to a marked degree, in so far as its activity has been translated, for the most part, from the field of muscular activity to that of thought. That this is not altogether so, however, may be seen from the sands at Blackpool on August Bank Holiday, where actual physical contact seems to be the chief object. Nevertheless, what truly troubles man is not absence of this physical contact, so much as absence of mental and moral contact. In the next chapter, we shall have occasion to notice, how activities, which at lower levels proceed through engrams involving efferent paths to muscles and glands, are side-tracked into engrams comprising the great association areas of the brain which involve thought, the passage of activation to the muscular efferents being inhibited. So it is with the central nervous system neurones of this disposition, they are so conditioned, both in the cognitive and conative phase, that their relatedness is altered, but so far as the vegetative neurones are concerned, there is no such alteration in the engram, and so the affect remains much the same, whether the lack of contact is physical or mental.

A disposition described by McDougall as the instinct of appeal, is specially characteristic of gregarious animals. This would seem to be rather a new type of behaviour, emerging from primitive panic and primitive anger, rather than a fully organized independent instinct, for it comes into play when the animal is distressed or thwarted, especially in its efforts at flight or aggression. In this conation we meet with a true emergent, something quite new in behaviour, the uttering of a cry or noise. This new emergent in the process of mental evolution is of the very greatest importance; for, from the differentiation of this cry, is derived language and all that it involves.

The two remaining instincts which are to be discussed are of considerable moment, since they are the direct manifestations of the two biological principles on which life depends, namely the maintenance of the individual and the maintenance of the race.

The first, the food-seeking disposition, does not require much discussion here, since it is an organization on a higher level of the appetites of hunger and thirst, modified according to the requirements of the animal, according to its species, and its necessity to seek and perhaps kill its food. With this is related the acquisitive disposition, with its dual conations of collecting and hoarding. This is clearly derived primarily from the appetites of hunger, and is only secondarily transferred to other objects unconnected with food.

The second, the mating disposition, merits further discussion. In animals, this disposition has for its end the biological function of perpetuation of the race, and is a higher organization of sexual appetite. In the majority of cases, it is not only confined to the period of life when the animal is full grown, and therefore capable of performing this important function to the best advantage, but also to special periods of varying length and frequency, termed oestral cycles, to which the active exhibition of this behaviour is limited. In man on the other hand, though the active period is more or less confined to the years during which he is full grown, once sexual activity has started, there is no periodic interruption at all. Perhaps associated with this prolongation of the opportunities for sexual activity, we find that man does not only use this disposition to fulfil its biological function, but also for the purposes of obtaining pleasure for himself. This latter function is only possible at the level of self-consciousness and reflective thought, for though pleasure may be gained incidentally in the course of various activities, it cannot be deliberately sought and schemed for, except at the higher levels. This mating impulse is clearly differentiated from the other similar dispositions, which have been under discussion, in a way analogous to the suckling reflex and parental dispositions. In the latter we saw that the conative phase involved the giving of something from the ego to another. But in addition to their centrifugal character, the sex appetite and derivative mating impulse involve behaviour which results in the creation of something quite new, the offspring. The characteristic, therefore, of this engraphic pattern is its creative function.

This creative conation is also seen in one other disposition, which is generally referred to as the constructive instinct. This is very well established in certain animals, especially in the insects, spiders and birds. In mammals it is much less defined, except in the case of the beavers; and in the primates any defined instinctive behaviour of this sort is conspicuous by its absence, though in man it persists as a diffuse impulse to make things. In its original form this constructive instinct is very closely bound up with sex, the construction invariably being to house the products of sexual conation. Unquestionably the behaviour incident in the parental disposition takes place in the constructed nest, but the making of nests and pairing are associated together, not the making of nests and rearing the young. Moreover both are preparatory to, and lead up to, the exhibition of the parental disposition. Therefore, it may be taken, that mating and construction are, in their original form, most closely associated together; so closely as to suggest that one may be derived from the other or from an original creative impulse. If this is admitted, it must at once be allowed that the differentiation between the mating disposition and the constructive disposition appeared early, and by the time the level which we have been discussing is reached, they have evolved in different directions in many respects, and each has emerged as a concrete entity. Yet in certain respects they show marked similarities. Just as man has largely transferred the mating disposition away from its biological function to serve his own pleasure, so has he transferred the constructive disposition from its biological function of nest building, to minister to his pleasure. From this constructive impulse has arisen the whole of man's artistic creation, which, though it serves no useful biological function, is a requirement of the human race, comparable to all instinctive types of reaction. This, therefore, may explain why artistic expression is so universal and almost necessary to mankind, and why it is so closely related to sex in many respects. It has been said that transference of a conation to serve the end of man's pleasure is only possible at the level of self-consciousness and reflective thought; and this must be so, for it involves the possibility of a control of his destiny, which is the peculiar attribute of man. This does not involve free-will in the commonly accepted sense, but a freedom in virtue of organization and relatedness, whereby a pattern of behaviour related to the self, as opposed to the environment, can serve as a stimulus for a further pattern of behaviour and so modify the whole constitution of the relationship of the ego and his surroundings. But this will be discussed more fully in Chapter XVII. Another aspect of the sex and mating disposition must be referred to, namely the inherent bivalency of the disposition. The balance between giving and taking in love relationship should be a nice one, and this seems to depend on the constitution of the sex appetite, upon which mating, and, at a higher level, love depend. Mention has already been made of this, when it was pointed out, that in addition to the appetition there was an expulsive pattern involved in the constitution of the appetite, which implies a definite bivalency of taking (appetition) and giving (expulsion). In love and the derivative relationships of friendship, these opposites do not always appear in the same proportions, but there is always an element of creative unselfish giving, and an element of destructive selfish taking. The creative generous lover is familiar, but so is the selfish and destructive vampire, and we may meet with all grades between the two extremes.

With this we have concluded the review of the more important dispositions with which man is equipped at birth. It remains to discuss how this organization of mental function continues, by means of growth and contact with the environment, until the complete personality emerges.

CHAPTER VII

THE FURTHER ORGANIZATION OF MENTAL FUNCTION

IT has already been pointed out that every mental process presents three phases for discussion, cognitive, affective and conative. Up to the present we have examined them together in the processes under discussion, giving to each a more or less equal value, but in the more complicated grades of mental development, which take place during the life of the individual, it is more convenient to examine the organization of what we may call affective or emotional processes, cognitive or thought processes, and conative processes or sentiments. Nevertheless, we must remember that these terms are only conveniences, and that there can be no real separation of the three phases.

The emotions—simple, compound and derived—constitute the more complicated affective processes—and we call them affective processes, because the most obvious feature of their organization is feeling. None the less, the term emotion only has a meaning, in virtue of the organization of affect with a definitely recognizable cognition, and a definitely recognizable "wish" for action. For example, we cannot be said to feel the emotion of curiosity, unless we can recognize a stimulus in the form of some strange object, and without experiencing an impulse to some sort of action in relation to it.

The nature and possible modifications of this conation or impulse to action, when organized on the fully conscious level, are somewhat different from those we have so far considered. At the level of instinct and emotional disposition, conation was defined as the mental correlate of the activation of the efferent division of the engram, which led to muscular activity, so that the efferent organization was essentially neuromuscular. Therefore if I felt curiosity at this level, I necessarily experienced an impulse to investigate the object of that curiosity. At the level of reflective thought, however, we have a more complex organization, and this would seem to involve a redistribution of the efferent activity or, expressed from the psychological standpoint, a new orientation of the conation. With the great complication of the arrangement of neurones at this high level, which is characteristic of man, the possible "motor paths," open for activation, are enormously increased. So far, the efferent activation has typically served as the stimulus to muscular activity, the activation passing to a peripheral motor nerve, after traversing a limited number of intermediate central neurones. At the higher level however, the activation may be side-tracked to other engrams in the higher areas of the brain, so that it passes through to further intermediate central neurones, and may never influence a peripheral motor nerve so as to induce muscular activity. Thus the process may go on, from engram to engram, through the newer anatomical structures of the "association areas," without involving overt behaviour, though it does involve a psychological function, namely thought. Such activation would seem to be accompanied by the new emergent, which we call reflective thought. In this process, every efferent conation of one engram, becomes immediately an afferent cognition for the next, and hence thought is a development on the cognitive side, and, by reason of the cortical functions of integration and discrimination, one thought can be compared with another. This statement, however, requires qualification. We have said that the process of activation of neurones in the higher areas, described above, does not involve muscular action ; but this is not strictly true. The Behaviourist school has rightly pointed out that thought is accompanied by minute, scarcely observable muscular movements, of lips, tongue, larynx, eyes and so on. They go on to say that this is thought, and where such movements are not apparently present, such absence is due merely to difficulties of observation. This is a presumption, which we are hardly prepared to follow. We have argued above, that feeling is the mental correlate of the activation of certain vegetative neurones, and it seems reasonable to suppose that thought may be the mental correlate of the activation of cognitive neurones in the higher realms of the cortex. But we cannot prove this thesis ; nor can the Behaviourists prove that thought is the function of those minute muscular movements. However, it does not seem that the issue is of great practical importance. It is sufficient to say that these minute muscular movements do accompany certain thought processes, though they are not necessarily causative. Perhaps the most plausible explanation may be as follows. We have said that reflective thought involves activation of large numbers of intermediate neurones, accompanied by an inhibition of activation of neuromuscular patterns. Such inhibition is not always absolute, but may be relative, so that some part of the activation may be able to pass the resistance of the synapses, and activate the neuromuscular patterns in a feeble way. As Janet[1] has pointed out, the higher the level of cortical organization, the more efficiency is attained, but the violence of activity is lessened. For instance, compare the movement of the limb in voluntary activity, with that during an epileptic fit. According to this law, the higher the level of thought, the less activation will proceed through the neuromuscular pattern, since the new engrams will be more efficiently established, and the inhibitions more complete. This is borne out by the fact that when the savage or the child thinks, the process is very apt to be accompanied by observable, or even comparatively violent muscular movements of silent speech or gesticulation; and further, when we are excited, that is to say, when the general control of our mental processes is lessened, we are apt to make muscular movements of which we are quite unaware, but which are quite evident even to the casual observer. This merely illustrates the fact that, though the neural mechanisms which subserve conation may not be so obvious in thought processes, as they are when muscular action ensues, they are none the less present. Thus, when we feel curiosity, though we may not approach the object to investigate it, but may sit and ponder over the possibilities, nevertheless conation does occur and forms part of the process. Similarly, when we consider the organization of cognitive processes into perceptions, apperceptions and beliefs, all these involve conation in the sense we have discussed.

In the same way, thought always involves affect. It is sometimes held that reflecting upon a mathematical problem is not accompanied by feeling. But this cannot be the case, as the reflection on such a problem is not an isolated event, which can be plucked out of its content. It is all part of a process and is related to some sentiment, probably to that of the piece of work in hand, or to the self-regarding sentiment, which must involve feeling, as we shall see later when we study sentiments. Moreover, no process of thought, however abstract, can be entirely divested of such emotions as curiosity, hope, despondency, elation and so on. Thought, therefore, can never be divorced from affect, any more than it can be from conation. Again, the organization of conations into sentiments and character, involves a cognitive recognition of the object of the sentiment, and quite definite feeling towards it. Hence, although, for convenience, we talk about organization of these various phases, we do not depart from the general structure which we have laid down as essential to mental processes, but merely lay stress on the greater significance of one phase or the other, in the process under examination.

In a discussion of the organization of affective reactions, we cannot do better than follow McDougall, as we have, to a large extent, done so far. We must however insist that, as the primary emotional dispositions involve engraphic arrangements of neurones in the nervous system, so, the more complex psychical organizations involve more complex physical organizations, always remembering that any given neurone, far from having any correlation with any given mental "element," may be a constituent in any number of engrams, just as in our previously quoted analogy, any given stretch of railway line might figure in any number of routes from place to place, as laid down in the railway timetables of the country. Further, it is postulated that the various emotional experiences, so far as affect is concerned, are the mental correlates of various combinations of the sensory patterns, depending on tensions in the visceral field.

When the emotional dispositions, previously discussed, are organized on the cortical level of full consciousness, so that we are aware of the object of our emotion, and have control and discrimination of the subsequent conation, we may describe them as true emotions. In addition, we find the simple emotions combined in certain ways so that new compound emotions emerge. But it must be pointed out that the emergents described by McDougall as the compound emotions, are not the only ones possible, but that the same simple emotions may combine and emerge as something quite different. These atypical emergents are usually associated with some pathological state of mental function, whether instability, dissociation, or retardation, and very often they cannot be given a name; but, having drawn attention to this, we need not concern ourselves further with this matter here. Considerations of space forbid a full discussion of the compound emotions, and reference must be made to McDougall's[2] work for this purpose. However, we may quote his treatment of the compound emotion of reverence, to illustrate the sort of integration which takes place. Admiration is certainly a true emotion, and is, as certainly, not primary. It is distinctly a complex affective state, and implies a considerable degree of mental development. We can hardly suppose any of the animals to be capable of admiration, in the proper sense of the word, nor is it displayed by very young children. It is not merely a pleasurable perception or contemplation. One may get a certain pleasure from the perception or contemplation of an object without feeling any admiration for it—e.g., a popular ditty played on a barrel-organ may give one pleasure though one admires neither the ditty, nor the mode of its production, and though one may despise oneself a little, on account of the pleasure one feels. Nor is it merely intellectual and pleasurable appreciation of the greatness or excellence of the object. There seem to be two primary emotions essentially involved in the complex state provoked by the contemplation of the admired object, namely, wonder, and negative self-feeling or the emotion of submission. Wonder is revealed by the impulse to approach, and to continue to contemplate the admired object; for, as we saw, this is the characteristic impulse of the "instinct" of curiosity, and wonder is clearly expressed on the face, in intense admiration. In the admiration of older children, one may observe wonder very clearly expressed and dominant. 'Oh, how wonderful!' or 'Oh, how clever!' or 'How did you do it?' are phrases in which a child naturally expresses its admiration, and by which the element of wonder and the impulse of curiosity are clearly revealed. But, as soon as we feel that we completely understand the object we have admired, and can wholly account for it, our wonder ceases, and the emotion evoked by it is no longer admiration.

But admiration is more than wonder. We do not simply

proceed to examine the admired object, as we should one that provokes merely our curiosity or wonder. We approach it slowly, with a certain hesitation; we are humbled by its presence, and in the case of a person whom we intensely admire, we become shy, like a child in the presence of an adult stranger; we have the impulse to shrink together, to be still, and to avoid attracting his attention; that is to say, the instinct of submission, of self-abasement, is excited, with its corresponding emotion of negative self-feeling, by the perception that we are in the presence of a superior power, something greater than ourselves.

As an example of the further complication of emotion, let us consider the nature of our emotion, if the object that excites our admiration is also of a threatening or mysterious nature, and therefore, capable of exciting fear: e.g., a tremendous force in action, such as the Victoria Falls, or the display of the aurora borealis, or a magnificent thunder-storm. The impulse of admiration to draw near humbly, and to contemplate the object is more or less neutralized by an impulse to withdraw, to run away, i.e., the impulse of fear. We are kept suspended in the middle distance, neither approaching very near, nor going quite away; admiration is blended with fear, and we experience the emotion we call awe.

Awe is of many shades, ranging from that in which admiration is but slightly tinged with fear, to that in which fear is but slightly tinged with admiration. Admiration is, then, a binary compound, awe a tertiary compound. And awe may be further blended to form a still more complex emotion. Suppose that the power that excites awe is also one that you have reason to regard as beneficent, one that, while capable of annihilating us in a moment, yet works for our good, sustains and protects us, one that evokes gratitude. Awe then becomes compounded with gratitude, and we experience the highly compound emotion of reverence. This is the religious emotion par excellence; few merely human powers are capable of exciting reverence, this blend of wonder, fear, gratitude and negative self-feeling. Those human beings who inspire reverence, or who are by custom and convention considered to be entitled to inspire it, usually owe their reverend character to their being regarded as the ministers and dispensers of divine power.

What then is gratitude, which enters into the emotion

of reverence for the divine power? Gratitude is itself complex. It is a binary compound of tender emotion and negative self-feeling. To this view it may be objected that if tender emotion is the emotion of the parental instinct, whose impulse is to protect, how can this emotion be evoked by the divine power? The answer to this question is that it is evoked in the same way as the child's tender emotion towards the parent is evoked, namely by sympathy. The other element in gratitude is that negative self-feeling, which is evoked by the sense of the superior power of another. The act that is to inspire gratitude must make us aware, not only of the kindly feeling, the tender emotion of the other towards us; it must also make us aware of his power, and we must see that he is able to do for us something that we cannot do for ourselves. The element of negative self-feeling, then, is blended with tenderness in true gratitude, and its impulse, the impulse to withdraw from the attention of, or to humble oneself in the presence of its object, more or less neutralizes the impulse of the tender emotion to approach its object; the attitude typical and symbolical of gratitude is that of kneeling to kiss the hand that gives. Other compound emotions of this sort are pity, jealousy, shame and so forth; and as has been said, these emergents may be more manifold than we have names to give them.

The characteristic of these simple and compound emotions is that they occur in the organization of definite dispositions, with definite cognitive and conative phases of a permanent, though modifiable character. In other words they take their place as part of the function of a more or less permanent and specific engram. Given any one phase of these dispositions, the rest is predictable, as the emotion is always associated with a more or less definite situation. The derived emotions, on the other hand, may arise in the course of the activity of any of these dispositions. That is to say, that under certain circumstances, in the course of the activation of an engram, the neurones which subserve these derived emotions may be coincidently activated, but are not part of the original pattern as inherently laid down. For example, the sight of a sick child is associated with the emotion of pity, and the impulse to assist. That is the correlate of an engraphic activation inherently present in the architectural structure of the nervous system. However, in the course of this process, any of the derived emotions, hope, despair, anxiety and so on, may intervene. These are the correlates of activation of neurones, other than those which constitute definite inherent dispositions, and they do not tend to form permanent components of sentiments.

The derived emotions are met with at a level at which imagination, both prospective and retrospective, has come into play. These emotions divide themselves into a prospective group—confidence, hope, anxiety, despondency, despair—and into a retrospective group—regret, remorse and sorrow. A few others will be mentioned presently. To follow McDougall again, we may say that the derived emotions may occur in the course of any line of action, either singly or consecutively, depending for their intensity on the strength of the original conation; and in their turn contributing to the persistency of the conation. In this respect they are analogous to the effect of endocrine activity, in inducing a persistent effect of vegetative nervous activity; and doubtless their nature depends, to a large extent, on the state of the endocrine glands. For example, suppose I am setting out to climb a mountain, I awake early, the day is fine and I set out, full of confidence that I shall reach the top. Things may go perfectly smoothly, and the confidence persists until I have achieved my object. Or, I may find that the preliminary slopes are much more arduous than I expected, and instead of reaching the beginning of the real climb in two hours, I take three. By this time I am not so confident, but I am still full of hope, and go on with full determination to succeed. About half-way up, I notice that clouds are gathering very fast, and I know that the mountain is very dangerous in fog. I alternate between determination and expectancy that I shall succeed, and doubt and fear lest I shall fail, or even worse befall me. This "long drawn out fear" is anxiety. An hour later, I am still some hundreds of feet from the top when the fog closes down completely, and I realize that I shall never reach the top; so I give up the attempt, and sit down to rest in a state of despondency. Then I start to go down, still enveloped in fog, but I suddenly realize that I have lost my way, that I have eaten all my food, that no one knows exactly where I am. I reflect on all the disasters which have occurred on this mountain, and I give way to despair, in which state I cease to make any effort whatever.

When I have more or less recovered from this state of utter despair, and am sitting waiting for the mist to clear, I may carry my mind back, so to speak. I may then experience regret that I did not get up two hours earlier, or that I did not heed the warnings of the peasant I passed on the way, whom I had regarded as a miserable croaker. Then I may suddenly remember that I had left my dog shut up in a room, where he can get no food or drink, and I may reflect that I shall not get down to let him out for hours, or perhaps not at all, and I experience remorse. Upon this I settle down and think how I enjoyed life, how well I was getting on in my career, and I experience sorrow for myself. Then suddenly the mist clears, the sun comes out, I find that I am much nearer the bottom than I thought, and I experience joy, because I realize that I have got on better than I expected. Finally, while walking back towards home, I suddenly see my dog running towards me, whom I thought was shut up in the house, and I experience surprise. From this imaginary sequence of events, the reader may understand what is meant by the term derived emotions, and it is clear that they may occur in the course of any line of action.

It would seem that confidence is the correlate of the pleasurable sensory pattern, depending on tensions, or absence of tension accompanying an anticipated conation with no prospect of failure. Despair, on the other hand, is the correlate of the unpleasurable pattern of tensions accompanying an anticipated conation, with no prospect of success, while hope, anxiety, and despondency are emergents from various combinations of these. Regret is the retrospective reflection of failure, corresponding to the prospective tensions of despair. If regret involves a pattern which subserves something or someone for whom tender feeling is habitually experienced, whether self or some loved one, then sorrow is experienced. If to this, is added the high grade pattern of self-criticism, remorse is felt.

Joy is both retrospective and prospective. It accompanies imagination of success achieved, but particularly the retrospective aspect of this. Shand[8] regards joy as a definite disposition, and treats it at great length, but though a difficult subject, it seems to fit into the category of derived emotions more satisfactorily than into that of dispositions.

Surprise, as McDougall says, is more difficult to analyse, but it seems to be the correlate of that pattern of tensions which eventuates from a sudden intervention of a new stimulus, in the progress of a conation, at the level of prospective imagination and reflective thought, since, unless we have some sort of image of the expected end, we cannot experience surprise at its failure to eventuate.

Finally, amongst the affective organizations, we must consider belief and doubt. These processes essentially involve integration on the level of reflective thought. The animals cannot be said to believe or doubt. For example, suppose a young horse sees a strange object, he may alternately approach it, or retreat from it, because his behaviour is alternately in accordance with the pattern of his "curiosity" disposition and his "fear flight" disposition; but he does not doubt. The integration of the process has not reached that level. In order to doubt, I must have at least two questions on which I can reflect, Is this so? and Is it not so? We say that anxiety depends on affective correlates of tensions resulting from alternating prospective success or failure of conations. Doubt is an analogous affective experience, translated to the field of intellectual propositions, rather than simple conations. We may doubt in respect of a purely abstract intellectual proposition, for instance, as to whether men live on Mars, or we may doubt as to what we are going to do in the next quarter of an hour; but in the latter case, if we are really to experience doubt, we must present possibilities of action to ourselves in the form of questions, am I to go to sleep? or, am I to go for a walk? These are discriminated and judged upon in the field of intellectual activity, and not in the field of conation, leading to overt behaviour. The affective experience of doubt then, accompanies the highest discriminative function of our cortex, namely judgment and reason, and is integrated at the highest levels of its development which subserve reflective thought. The affect would seem to be the unpleasurable correlate of the sensory pattern, derived from the visceral tensions, involved in the failure of the opposed patterns to achieve co-ordination. This state is an interesting example of the importance of the lowest visceral functions, co-ordinated with the highest cortical activity, and illustrates how all mental processes are a unity, and may involve and include the lower processes by fusion, without any suppression whatever.

Belief, similarly, is an organization of pleasurable affective patterns on the plane of reflective thought, and follows when the patterns between which judgment is made have been co-ordinated and resolved into a single proposition. The more perfect the co-ordination, the freer from unpleasurable tensions will the affective pattern be, and therefore, the "stronger" the belief. This refers to true logical belief at the highest level, which presupposes a state of doubt that has been resolved by what is called reasoning. However, the same pleasurable affective tensions exist implicitly at lower levels. Thus the proposition, "the world is flat," may be implicitly believed in by the illiterate peasant, because there is no evidence from his senses to contradict it. Hence there are no unpleasurable tensions from activation of opposing visceral patterns, which engender doubt. Later the illiterate begins to learn, and various phenomena are pointed out to him, which he had never noticed before. These give evidence that the world is not flat, his implicit belief is shaken, and he enters into a stage of doubt. From this experience of tension he is eventually relieved when, with the increase of his knowledge, he reaches a sufficiently high level of organization to form a judgment, and he can appreciate the conclusive evidence for roundness. His doubts are allayed and he again achieves the pleasurable affective state of firm belief.

Primarily therefore, the child experiences an affective state of implicit belief in respect to all propositions, whether submitted to him in the form of evidence from his own senses, or as suggestions from others. It is only with the growth of experience, knowledge and discriminative function, that he experiences doubt. In certain cases, this doubt is integrated once more into a unity which constitutes belief, with the growth of the higher functions which subserve judgments and reasoning, and the more beliefs that can be established, the more chance of stability of personality does he have. Before discussing this further, however, we must turn to the organization of cognitive processes.

When referring to Semon's Mnemic laws in Chapter II, we drew attention to the fact that once the various systems of neurones had been arranged engraphically, a similar stimulus pattern, or part of such pattern, as had already established the engram, was capable of reactivating the engram, so that its mental and physical correlates could again be experienced or observed. The mental aspects of such reactivations at the level of full consciousness, are what are known as images, and may involve visual activities, auditory activities, and so on. Images may be represented below the level of consciousness; but, for the purposes of this discussion, we propose to confine the term to the usually accepted meaning of re-presented sensory experiences, of which the subject is aware. The representation is more or less exact, though it never can be precisely so, since it involves a new relatedness. This recall of the more or less exact image of the original pattern, constitutes what Varendonck[4] has called reduplicative memory. This is characteristic of instinctive and habitual behaviour at, or below conscious level, in which the same engraphically determined pattern may be evoked again and again, as when the bee repeats the same geometrical structure of cell, time after time, or we follow the same routine in retiring to bed, night after night. It is also characteristic of the mental processes of children, primitives and retarded personalities. Moreover, it is used constantly in the everyday life of normal people, when exact representation is all that is required to serve the end of our behaviour. None the less, as these engrams become organized on the level of higher cortical function, this type of memory tends to give place to a different type, termed by Varendonck "synthetic memory." The latter depends on the discriminative and integrative functions of the cortex, which determine a certain combination of significant features in the re-presented pattern to form a new and more efficient emergence. This discriminative and selective function, is not confined to these higher cognitive processes, which subserve abstract and creative thinking, as some are disposed to argue, but is also met with in connexion with purely muscular and sensory activity. The highly differentiated movements of the fingers of the pianist, or the subtle discrimination of the palate of the wine taster, depend on the acquisition of higher cortical function of a similar nature to that which subserves synthetic memory. As higher levels of function are involved, the tendency is for the process to become apparently simpler, more efficient and less violent, and this characterizes the difference between synthetic and reduplicative memory. Side by side, with the development of these cortical functions, which permit of discrimination and selection, the cognitive processes of man have been advanced enormously by the growth of language. Names or tokens of certain sensory patterns seem to have been the fundamental origin of language, and these greatly simplify thought processes and the use of imagery. It will be remembered, that in discussing the inherent motor dispositions, we described the disposition of appeal. As McDougall[5] has suggested, this is probably the basis of language, since it is the only primary disposition, which has the production of voice as its conation. With increasing organization however, this conative pattern has been translated from its original purpose of a cry for help, to subserve functions in the organization of other impulses, specially in relation to mating, active sympathy and the gregarious "instinct"—the three specially socializing dispositions. This already lays down a differentiation of voice, in the call to the mate, the warning of danger, and so on. In the dog we can easily recognize differentiation of voice sounds, in the growl of anger, the yelp of food seeking, the whine of self-abasement, and the bark of pure excitement. In point of fact, this conation of voice production tends to become differentiated and organized in relation to the primary dispositions. It is easy to imagine further differentiation of voice sounds, say in the case of the warning cry of danger, whereby one sound meant lion, another snake and another tiger and so on. Thus we have established sounds, representing the names of things, which specially characterize the language of primitives. These races tend to name very general groups, such as trees, and then specific examples, and not generic classes, since the secondary synthetic power is not yet developed. Thus we have the example of aborigines, who have a name for tree and different names for all varieties of oak tree, but no name for the genus oak. Later, however, particulars become collected into more general groups, which makes for greater simplicity and efficiency in speech. From this the growth of language is not difficult to follow until it reaches the complexity of the modern civilized tongues. Having gained the power of selection among images and sensations and, by means of language, acquired a ready means of presenting them to ourselves or others, the next advance is the power of directing attention to such images or sensations. When referring to function at cortical level, we noted that the organization of engrams is such, that when any engraphic pattern is in action there is also in consciousness, a fading impression of the mental correlate of the engram, which has just preceded the one in action, and a somewhat dim forecast of the engram about to be activated. The condition of passive or implicit attention would seem to depend on the fact that the most definite activation is taking place in the engram, which is said to be in the focus of consciousness; the past and future engram being said to be in the margin of consciousness. Implicit attention is chiefly noticeable in the correlates of those engrams, whose stimulus pattern is most intense or most persistent. "Active" attention depends on the organization of engrams, or their correlated patterns, into systems with an affective appeal. These systems, complexes, or constellations, are in relation to one or more of our dominant sentiments. For instance, we can, as a rule, fix our attention on incidents or images in relation to our ambitions, our loves and hates, and it is in virtue of the organization of the pattern in relation to these sentiments, that the so-called fixation of attention is possible. Again, therefore, active attention depends on higher cortical function, and is an emergent, depending on a new relatedness. The succession of activation of engrams subserves the stream of consciousness, and allows for consecutiveness of thought. Also this allows for what we call prospective imagination, whereby we forestall actual behaviour by "imagining it in our mind's eye." Prospective imagination of something absolutely new and altogether outside our experience is impossible, for it necessarily involves the activation of an engram already laid down, but the selective and reintegrative function already referred to, allows for new groupings within the engram, so that a new emergent from old material may arise. Of such sort is the creative imagination of the artist and the genius. However, it is clear that such prospective imagination would be impossible were it not for the short cut provided by symbolic images of various sorts, and especially by language, for in this way the subject, working in imagination, escapes the necessity of having to go through the long tedious process of redintegration, but achieves results by selection and synthesis. This stream of prospective imagination is specially characteristic of dreams and phantasy formation, which are not subjected to the control of the higher forms of thought, termed reasoning, and are never interrupted by muscular activity.

To return to the activation of engrams, imagination depends on the spread of activity through a series of these, and with each a mental correlate will be experienced, having an organization related to that of the engram. The nature of our most ordinary mental experiences is not only dependent on the exact representation of the engraphic correlates, but will depend on several other factors, amongst which are the effects of the present stimulus, the organization of past engraphic effects, certain facilitations and inhibitions, depending on temporary temperamental factors, and so on. Each such experience—or perception—is a true emergent, something coherent in itself, having its own organization and form. This is what the Gestalt theory seeks to demonstrate, that perceptions are not mere agglomerations of sensations and images but have a definite form and structure of their own and are recognized in consciousness, in virtue of that form and structure, and acquire meaning only in virtue of this inherent organization. Hence, part of a perception is meaningless, and is incapable of being considered in consciousness, since the very essential nature of the perception is its wholeness. A perception from its very nature is necessarily conscious, and, except as an emergent whole, it cannot attain that relatedness which involves consciousness. This essential structure and form is not hard to grasp, if a perception is considered as the correlate of an engram, organized at the level of full cortical function, where a very definite degree of integration has been reached. This factor of form is another means whereby mental processes are simplified at higher levels, and we come across it again and again all the way up to the thought of the physicist and mathematician, who frequently helps himself by constructing images of organized form, and the artist who composes his picture in relation to forms and volumes. This organization into complex, but yet integrated form, has only been recently recognized, for it was obscured by the much discussed process of association. This constitutes a linking together of engraphic patterns, with their correlates, the perceptions, by some of the many ties described by the association psychologists; but this linking together only becomes significant when it leads to a new organization. In itself, the mere process of association, independently of the essential higher functions of the cortex, may occur in the incoherence of dreams and the redintegrations of the insane, and has no significance.

The primary perceptions of the child and the primitive are generic rather than particular, and the first advance is by the function of discrimination. Consider the child's impression of any presentation of its environment. Certain of these presentations appear to him as four-legged moving beings. These are then discriminated into bow-wows, pussies, and so on, depending on his auditory and other simple sensory impressions. Gradually, as this formal perception is enriched by experience, suggestion and instruction, he is enabled to discriminate between the various sorts of bow-wow, till he can differentiate almost any variety. On this process of discrimination, combined with the opportunities of experience and instruction enjoyed by the subject, depends the acquisition of knowledge. Personalities vary greatly in this power of discrimination, and consequently of acquiring knowledge, but they vary still more in the higher functions which involve the application of knowledge. It is clear, that if this process of discrimination was to continue indefinitely, the individual would be provided with an enormous number of separate perceptions, whose very multiplicity would lead to confusion and futility. Hence the next process is a re-synthesis of individual perceptions into general classes, grouped according to significant features. This process is termed apperception, and involves the formation of concepts. For example, suppose a child uninstructed in physics has regarded ice, water, and steam as essentially different substances, having nothing to do with each other. Then he learns, that, if subjected to a sufficiently high temperature, ice first becomes water, and then steam; and that steam sufficiently cooled becomes first water, and then ice; and similarly water, subjected to the proper conditions, may be converted into either ice, or steam, he realizes that they are, in fact, the same substance under different physical forms. This grouping of these three separate perceptions into one, which may further be symbolized under the sign H_2O, obviously allows for short cuts in thought, and enormously simplifies the engraphic pattern.

Apparently in certain people at any rate, this grouping

of perceptions by appreciation of common features, may go on below the level of conscious awareness, in which case, the new emergent structure appears in the form of an intuition. With the emergence of concepts we find a further organization with the affective patterns, which have been referred to as belief. The simpler concepts may give rise to conflict, and engender doubt, or be further integrated and give rise to more general beliefs, and this leads to the next step in the organization of cognitive dispositions by the process of reasoning. The functions of discrimination and apperception, on the level of reflective thought, allow us to present for consideration propositions which are correlates of complicated engrams, which involve the pleasurable patterns subserving the affect of belief. In the process of reasoning the functions of discrimination and integration come into play at the highest level. The simplest form of reasoning is from two particular beliefs to a third. Thus, experience tells us that steam is hotter than water, and there being no counter experience to engender doubt, this proposition is accompanied by belief. Secondly, experience establishes a further belief that water is hotter than ice. Therefore reason tells us that steam is hotter than ice. Such an example of reasoning is so crude as to savour of the ridiculous, but it serves as an example of a large class of mental processes whereby new beliefs are formed and knowledge is applied. They may be expressed by the formula $X = Y$ and $Y = Z \therefore Z = X$. This form of reasoning is simple, and gives rise to reliable propositions.

The next step is inductive reasoning. This consists of the argument from the particular to the general, which may be exemplified by the following example. I have seen and touched a very large number of fish, and all these are cold-blooded, therefore all fish are cold-blooded. This type of argument is extremely common, and is very useful for arranging facts, but its inherent possibility of fallacy must be remembered. For example, it is possible, however improbable it may be, that one day I might come across a warm-blooded fish, when the whole argument would fall to the ground. The possible fallacy of such reasoning is more apparent from such an example as the following. Suppose I have to catch a train every morning, and for months it is at least five minutes late, it is a legitimate inductive argument that I can always take five minutes more over breakfast; but one day I shall certainly miss my train. Hence, a belief established by inductive reasoning should never be so organized as to be essential to the stability of the personality, for it is always liable to be upset. The form of argument of inductive reasoning may be represented thus:

$$X = Y,\ X_1 = Y,\ X_2 = Y,\ X_n = Y,\ \therefore \text{ all } X\text{'s} = Y.$$

The third type of reasoning is known as deductive reasoning, and is an argument from the general to the particular. This may be exemplified as follows. I am walking on a tableland, from which I wish to descend. I come to a stream flowing westwards. I argue, water always flows down hill, this water is flowing westwards, therefore westwards is dowr. hill. This type of argument is dependable, provided the premises are reliable, but if not, then the most grievous errors may be arrived at by the most logical processes, as may be seen in the delusions of certain insane persons—the paranoiacs. This form of argument may be represented by the formula:—all X's are Y's, Z is an X. ∴ Z is a Y, but the fallacy expressed thus, all X's are Y's, Z is a Y, ∴ Z is an X, must be carefully guarded against.

All these processes of reasoning result in systems of beliefs, which are of the greatest importance to the personality. When formulated in the realm of reality they are referred to as convictions of facts, but when they are formulated in the realms of phantasy, or ethics, they are referred to as faith. The freer these systems of belief are from the tensions engendered by doubt, the more stable will be the personality. Further, this stability will be achieved in so far as these various systems of belief are organized into a coherent philosophy of life. A spurious stability may be established if the systems which conflict with each other are kept in what have been termed logic-tight compartments, so that they are never allowed to become associated in such a way, that the tensions of doubt are engendered. For instance, it is not uncommon to find an employer of labour seriously denouncing the evils of slum dwellings, and pointing out how this leads to the ill-health and inefficiency of his work-people, while he gladly accepted the good rents from this class of real estate. Shaw has dramatized this situation in *Widowers' Houses*. Sooner or later, however, circumstances arise in most cases, which break down these artificial barriers and stability is seriously threatened, if not actually interfered with.

Personalities vary considerably in their capacity of exercising the higher functions of thought, which we may term intelligence, and consequently in the degree to which they can build up these systems of beliefs, and use them in the general organization of their minds.

Some people go through life with these systems unorganized into any definite structural whole, but they generally fail practically, since there is no unity in their personalities. They are sometimes said to have no beliefs, but only working hypotheses. This is not an accurate description, since it is not an absence of beliefs, but an absence of organization of beliefs, that is characteristic. In these people, the upsetting of any one system of belief has little or no effect on the rest, and so does not seriously affect the personality as a whole. At the other end of the scale are those people whose beliefs are all narrowly integrated together, so that the whole structure stands or falls by each separate system. These tend to weave their philosophy of life into a sentiment, without due regard to a comprehensive relationship with the environment; that is to say the integration of this philosophy of life is at a lower level than the general organization of the self-regarding sentiment to which we shall refer presently. In this process of integration all sorts of emotional dispositions are centred round the philosophy professed. This state may be exemplified by the extreme Puritan, who hated and feared those that disagreed with his creed, was elated if he felt that his behaviour upheld it, loved those who professed it, and so on. The most desirable personality is presumably he in whom there is a well organized system of beliefs, constituting a satisfactory philosophy of life. This philosophy of life should not be too unyielding and narrow, but should be comprehensive and capable of modification within its own structure.

Finally, we must consider the organization of conative processes. First of all, it will be as well to draw attention to the fact that we are dealing with purely mental processes, and to guard against the fallacy of loose terms, which imply that a conation, or any other mental process, can do anything. There is only one source of energy in the body, and that is provided by the combustion of fuel, which in living organisms takes the form of digestion of the food. To take an analogy, a motor car can do nothing by itself, it can only work by means of the combustion of petrol; but the car will go faster and more efficiently on the same amount of petrol if all its parts are properly fitted together, and all its nuts and screws are tight, also if all sources of internal friction are removed. Similarly with conations, if the patterns on which they depend are firmly organized, and so constituted that the whole efferent tract to the final motor path, whatever it may be, is facilitated, and free from inhibitions, the resulting activity will be more efficient. Therefore, when we say this conation, impulse, urge, or whatever we call it, is stronger or more vigorous than that other, all we mean is that the pattern through which the efferent activation progresses, is better organized and facilitated. The patterns, moreover, which are most closely organized and facilitated, are those which we have described as the primary emotional dispositions, and we find that when conation appears most vigorous, the pattern of behaviour is in accordance with one of these primary dispositions, fear, anger, curiosity, sex and the like.

This gives us means to understand such factors as interest and desire. We saw that passive implicit attention depended on the full activation of any particular engram. Active, so called voluntary, attention depends on the fact that the particular engram is organized with one of the primary dispositions, generally curiosity in the intellectual sphere, but also with others, and built up with a sentiment. Further, it is the conation, the wish, the urge, organized on the conscious level, which gives us the sense of effort, which we call "taking an interest." Similarly with desire, which is generally applied to the sphere of action, and not so much to the sphere of intellect. This is the mental correlate of another somewhat different organization of the conative pattern on the conscious level, and the urgency of desire depends on the closeness with which the engram under activation is organized with one of the primary dispositions, or built up within a definite sentiment and the degree of facilitation within this engram. To go back to our analogy of the network of railway lines, we may suppose that at various parts, there were stretches of line, particularly well laid, particularly smooth and frictionless, which would correspond to the primary dispositions. The rest varied very considerably in its quality, some being very poorly put together, with frequent unevenness and friction. It is clear, that given a constant fuel consumption, the more the train could run over the smooth parts in going from any one place to any other place by the scheduled routes, the more speed, efficiency and apparent power it would exhibit, but this power would only be apparent, for it depends on the permanent way, and not on the fuel consumption of the engine.

In discussing the organization of conative dispositions, we cannot do better than follow McDougall again in his conceptions of the sentiments. A sentiment may be defined, as an organization of affective dispositions in relation to an object, so that the various conative trends are modified in relation to this object. The object may be anything at all, animate or inanimate, work, golf, or child, and the organization of conative dispositions will depend on the nature of the sentiments. Examples of sentiments are love, hate, contempt, respect, friendship and so on, but it is evident that the combination may be legion, and for many of the emergents we can have no name. As an example, we may indicate how the dispositions are organized within the sentiment of love. Self-abasement is felt in the presence of the loved one, who is generally felt as "far too good". Self-assertion is felt at having won such a prize, and at being thought worthy to love such a one. This is directed towards other people more than to the object of the love, and yet to a certain extent to the loved one as well. Fear is felt lest any danger should approach, anger against any that interfere with our relationship with the loved one, and also against any that should harm or threaten her. Tender emotion is felt in a desire to cherish and protect her, curiosity to find out all about her, and all sides of her character. One is open to suggestion from her and about her, one sympathizes with her and tends to imitate her actions, and throughout all is the strongly organized, and therefore conatively vigorous, mating impulse. These and other dispositions are all organized round the object of the loved one, and the more firmly organized the sentiment the "stronger" is the love. The more the relatively simple, closely organized, facilitated disposition of sex is dominant, especially if it is in its relatively low state of integration of appetite, the more "violent" will be the love, in accordance with the principle, that has been referred to before, that the higher the integration the more efficient, but less violent is the resultant pattern of behaviour. Hence, it may be seen that all sorts of variations may occur in the ultimate nature of a sentiment, according to the variation and proportion of the dispositions, which are organized within it; but this very organization will determine the conations and overt behaviour of the individual.

With the development of self-consciousness it necessarily follows that a strong, enduring and important sentiment must be formed round this new object, the self. This McDougall has termed the self-regarding sentiment, and, according to the organization and form of this will be determined all the relationships between the self and the environment in the widest sense. The sentiment will vary with the dominance of fear, curiosity, tender emotion and so on. Moreover this sentiment must necessarily embrace all others, love, hate, contempt, respect, friendship, and so on, for all sorts of objects, for they cannot exist except in relation to the self, and must be organized round the self.

We have now reached the point when we can consider the final organization which results in the emergence of the unique complete personality. This final organization would seem to be the union of the self-regarding sentiment with the philosophy of life, described above, as the provisional culmination of the cognitive dispositions, together with the all-important temperamental factor already discussed. This organization may help to explain how it is we can resist the common temptations of life, which seem to be so much more violent than what we call our moral sentiments. In spite of this violence however, if this new organization within the personality is firmly knit, then it will gather within its formal structure all these "lower" impulses so that they cannot "break loose and act on their own," unless the stability of organization weakens, and dissociation occurs. Let us take an analogy; imagine a highly trained organized troop of cavalry executing a musical ride; their coherence depends on the close and carefully organized form of the whole, and as this form alters and shifts in the course of the ride it presents kaleidoscopic changes to the onlooker, but always remains the same organized group, which may seem incapable of acting separately. But supposing discipline and control is relaxed over the individual rider and horse, that individual is capable of executing the most violent independent movements, and throwing the whole into the most unutterable confusion. Let the individual rider and horse represent the "lower" impulses, and the organized troop, the properly integrated personality, and we see how "giving way to temptation" depends on the disorganization of personality, and why the lower impulse sometimes wins the day and sometimes loses, in the apparently unequal struggle. It would be just as sensible or foolish to ask why, in the course of a musical ride, any one horse does not always turn and gallop away to its stable and its oats, as to ask why, in a well-organized personality, one of the lower impulses does not always become dominant, and stampede the personality in the direction of lust, theft, murder or panic. To push our analogy a little further, we may observe that the musical ride may be beautiful or ugly, efficient or untidy, according to the "form" in which it is organized. We have seen how important this "form" is, in relation to cognitive integration, and now we see that it is the philosophy of life which gives form to our behaviour, and determines the coherence and nature of the self-regarding sentiment. Before leaving this analogy however, it must be pointed out that it is not exact, and yet it may stand as an illustration. It is not exact, because the individual horse in the troop does have a separate source of energy belonging to its own individuality, which we cannot allow to the primary dispositions. The analogy would perhaps be closer, if we imagined the troop to be mechanical and coupled together, all driven by the same steam engine. But under certain conditions the couplings might break, and the individual units proceed to disintegrate the whole by their own momentum.

The philosophy of life, which we have described as the pattern according to which behaviour is determined, may be noble or ignoble, according to purely hedonistic principles of avoidance of pain and gaining of pleasure; according to the dictates of the eleventh commandment "thou shalt not be found out"; or according to the highest ideals and aspirations, of which the human race is capable. Our behaviour will be shaped in relation to this form of our philosophy, and hence the importance of having *some* philosophy of life, preferably a good one, with which our self-regarding sentiment may be integrated. Only so can we reach the desired end of the development of our personality, namely stability of structure, capable of modification within that structure so as to ensure adequate adjustment to the changing circumstances of the environment.

CHAPTER VIII

VARIATIONS IN PERSONALITIES

As far as space will allow, we have now completed the review of the scheme according to which we conceive the development of personality from the inherent dispositions, and have arrived at a point when we can consider the organized emergent as a whole.

So far, however, we have not laid sufficient stress on the influence of environment in moulding the personality. It is obvious that from the very moment of birth, environment as a whole influences and modifies the dispositions, and it is clearly impossible to follow out, in any general way, what must necessarily be an individual experience. However, there are certain environmental factors which require mention. To begin with, there are the physical factors in the environment, which may be grouped under the general term climatic. Next the generic factor, race, though not itself environmental, is involved in the acquired factor of social heritage. It is by no means an easy task to differentiate the particular contributions of these factors in the make-up of the individual, for no very accurate observations, on a sufficiently large scale, have been carried out. However, there is no doubt that there is a lot of truth in the popular conception that those who live in a cold bracing climate are on the whole more alert, more progressive, and more aggressive, than those who live in a warm relaxing climate. The latter tend to be inert, conservative, and prone to follow the path of least resistance. In these days of rapid communication, it is probably becoming increasingly hard to be certain of the exact influence of climate, for, in order to produce their effect, these physical factors must exert their influence continually and for some considerable time, and we are apt to attribute to "a change of air," effects which are due to quite different causes. If we have the misfortune to live and work in a relaxing climate we know the effect of the change to the sea or the hills, how our mind clears, how new apperceptions are achieved, and all our mental functions work at a higher level. All this we are apt to attribute, to the climatic change, forgetting the effect of freedom from worry, and fatigue, and the new stimulus patterns which are presented to our senses quite independently of changes of climate. Nevertheless, the fact remains, that any personality does have a climatic medium in which both physical and mental functions are at their best, and this varies with the individual. For instance, for one person the optimum is a mountain climate over 5000 feet, while others would feel no energy at all at such a height, indeed a case may be cited of a lady who is depressed by mountains to such an extent that she is acutely miserable while the train passes through Switzerland on the way to Italy, but quite regains her spirits on reaching the plain at Milan. McDougall[1] sums up the effects of climate as follows: "There is a fair consensus of opinion to the effect that what we may call climate exerts an important influence. In climate, the two factors recognized as of chief importance, are temperature and moisture. High temperature combined with moisture, certainly tends to depress the vital activity of Europeans, and to render them indolent and indisposed to exertion of any kind. On the other hand, high temperature combined with dryness of the atmosphere, seems to have the effect of rendering men but little disposed to continuous activity, and yet capable of great efforts; it tends to produce a violent, spasmodic activity. A cold climate seems to dispose towards sustained activity, and, when combined with much moisture, to a certain slowness. These effects, which we ourselves experience, and which we see produced upon other individuals on passing from one climate to another, we seem to see impressed upon many of the races, which have long been subjected to those climates; for example, the slow and lazy Malays have long occupied the hottest, moistest region of the earth. The Arabs and the fiery Sikhs, may be held to illustrate the effect of dry heat. The Englishman and the Dutchman show the effects of a moist cool climate, a certain sluggishness, embodied with great energy and perseverance." He quotes a somewhat doubtful example of more definitely physical modifications. Thus, it is said that in North America, a race characterized by a new specific combination of mental and physical qualities is being rapidly formed; and it seems to be well established that long slender hands are among these features; for in Paris, a specially long slender glove is made every year in large quantities for the American market. Again, we see apparently a change of physical type in the white inhabitants of Australia. They seem to be becoming taller and more slender—'cornstalks'; and this modification is commonly regarded as the direct effect of climate. That a new race or sub-race, with a specific combination of qualities, should be forming in America, is certainly to be expected from the fact that the intimate blending of a number of European stocks has been going on for some generations. But what gives special support to the assumption that these new qualities are the direct effects of climate, is that these physical qualities, at least, seem to be approximations to the type of the Red Indians, the aboriginal inhabitants. And, it is said, this approximation of type can only be due to hereditary accumulation of the direct effects of the climate on individuals. This, however, leads us on to the vexed question of inheritance of acquired characters, with which there is no space to deal here.

When we turn to the influence of race on the personality, we are met with the most perplexing problems. All through history many attempts have been made to differentiate racial characteristics and in modern times, since Jung[2] expounded his introvert and extravert types, many writers have tried their hand at differentiating the types, as exemplified by the various races. The difficulty in such work is that, even with scientific writers of the highest repute, the patriotic prejudices engendered by the late war, are not without their effect. Trotter's[3] efforts to classify nations in correspondence with animal herds, was not particularly happy, and the later efforts of McDougall,[4] Hinkle[5] and Seligman,[6] though full of interest and suggestion, are not altogether convincing. The fact of the matter is, that in any given race, there are so many exceptions that no rule can be satisfactorily established. For this reason no attempt will be made here to discuss the question of racial differences, since this belongs rather to the science of anthropology. It is sufficient to point out that racial differences do exist, and that however similar their climatic, social and educational environment, the respective descendants of Shem, Ham and Japheth can never emerge as identical personalities.

The next factor is what Mr Graham Wallas[7] has termed "social heritage." This corresponds, in some measure, to what Trotter calls the "herd instinct." The latter discusses this, not so much as a reaction of the individual in virtue of an inherent instinct, but rather as the influence of the attitude of the community on the individual. He shows how this attitude controls and restricts, not only the conations of man's primary dispositions, but also man's progress towards higher rational levels. In the last chapter it was assumed that the philosophy of life, which subserved the highest emergence, should be organized on the highest rational level, but it must be admitted at once, that this is not attained in the majority of cases. Our most fixed beliefs are too often merely the products of the suggestion of the community, and this especially applies to such as relate to our position in the universe and our object in life. The Christian and the Atheist, the Conservative and the Socialist, too often hold their beliefs because their set believe these doctrines, and not because they have arrived at their standpoint by any process of reasoning at all.

As a result of the possession of language and its derivatives, man has an enormous mass of this social heritage, which is the accumulated experience of the herds and communities into which the human race has been divided, but as Wallas points out, it is not confined to man. Zoologists have shown that many birds hand on individual experiences of song production, routes of migration, and habits of various sorts. For example the trick of getting at the kidneys of the sheep, which are their victims, seems to be a true social heritage of the mountain parrots of New Zealand, and the practice of sea-gulls flocking up the river to London in winter, was a habit engendered as recently as 1895, when a few gulls found refuge and food there, during an exceptionally prolonged cold spell. However, it is only in man that this social heritage has assumed such great importance. So great indeed is this, that it is doubtful if modern civilized man could long survive if deprived of all that it contributes to his daily life. The nature of this social heritage depends to a very large extent on the social class into which an individual is born, for this determines all sorts of important factors, both physical and mental. Obviously diet, fresh air, education and companionship are largely dependent on the social strata in which the child finds himself, but also, more subtle influences are thereby determined, such as the closeness of relationship with the parents and with brothers and sisters, the age at which the child has to enter the world and fend for himself, the degree of responsibility devolved upon him, both in respect of his younger brothers and sisters, and so on. In spite of these factors however, too much stress must not be laid on the influence of environment, for it is probable that much more is due to nature than to nurture, as may be seen by the very considerable variation amongst individuals of the same class and circumstances. For example, a statistical enquiry was made into the manual workers of Sheffield, some 800 men and women being taken for investigation. Of these it was found that 22 per cent. were of an exemplary type, sober, industrious and of sufficient intelligence to be worthy to exercise the vote; 14 per cent. were vicious and undesirable; while the remainder were of poor capabilities, incapable of advancing themselves in the world, and of barely sufficient intelligence to vote properly. It is possible that with a better social heritage this large middle group might have been improved, so as to be worthy of inclusion in the first group, but on the whole, they were condemned to hopeless mediocrity, by their lack of innate capabilities, rather than by their lack of opportunities.

Further elaboration of these environmental factors must be sought in works on anthropology and sociology, for it is impossible to discuss in any adequate way the infinite variety of environmental factors which influence the formation of personality, and we must be content to reiterate, that personality has no meaning in terms of nature alone, nor yet in terms of nurture alone, but is an emergent from the interrelatedness of the two.

It remains to consider broad factors determining the variations between personalities. In some cases grouped together under the head of retarded personalities, the individual is incapable of full development, owing to inherent defects of the nervous system. These merit separate discussion, in view of the light thrown by them on the development of the normal, and will be dealt with in Chapter XV. Others reach their full development abnormally early. Such are termed precocious. As has been seen already in Chapter V general precocity may be associated with anomalies of the endocrine system, but precocity in particular functions may also occur. Most, if not all individuals are provided with one or more talents, for instance for singing, for dancing, for construction, for abstract thought, and so on. These differ from the dispositions we have so far discussed, in being peculiar to the individual, and not general for the species. Everyone possesses an instinct, or emotional disposition of curiosity, but not everyone possesses a talent for singing. Such talents may be described as a special aptitude for some particular function, and these aptitudes depend on a specially organized engram, within which all neuronic connexions are facilitated; for it is noticeable that the activity represented by the talent is not only done well, but also easily and quickly. Talents are special developments of the functions we have learnt to regard as belonging to the highest levels of cortical activity. For example, the talented musician must be able to discriminate a variety of tones in such a way as to surpass the average person in the subtlety of this discrimination, so that he can distinguish, say, five separate tones, where the average man can only distinguish one. Then he must be capable of reintegration, so as to produce new tone combinations, and finally have such power of discriminative muscular movement as the technique of singing, piano-playing, or the like, demand. It is obvious that in the majority of cases such talents owe something to inherent dispositions, and a great deal to acquired skill, and the proportion of these two constituents will vary with the nature of the talent. In certain cases the talent appears precociously early in life, so that it is evident that the engram is almost entirely inherently constituted. The classical example is that of Mozart, who was able to play a piece on the piano at the age of three, with very little practice. It is to be noticed, however, as Darwin points out, that his action was not instinctive in the true sense. If this had been so, it must have resembled the duckling, which swims perfectly when put in the water, with no practice. None the less, as Ward[8] says, such precocious talents come remarkably close to instinctive action, and may eventually come to be instinctive, inasmuch as they can be performed without practice. Thus, if we accept at least the possibility of transmission of acquired characters, the talents of the present may represent the instincts of the future. Precocity of talents then, is an early organization and facilitation of certain engrams, subserving high-grade activity of considerable complexity. It is noticeable, however, that talents which are precocious are concerned with those levels of the cortex which are not of the very highest, but have to do with sensory and motor discrimination and integration, expressing themselves in terms of tone, colour and form. Hence we find precocity in music, painting and the manipulative arts, but not in abstract thought, or in the framing of philosophical concepts, since such function only comes to fruition later in life. Infant calculators are not uncommon, but probably this function has to do with perception of geometrical form, rather than with any real mathematical ability. Again reduplicative memory may be very highly developed at quite an early age, so that a young child may be able to repeat long passages by heart, but synthetical memory is not a feature that is ever to be met with till later.

While some personalities are retarded and others precocious, the majority develop up to a point, at much the same rate and in much the same way; but in the later stages of development there is a considerable difference in the extent of growth, and in the levels of so called intelligence which are reached. The intelligence of a person is not his intellectual knowledge, but his capacity for using that knowledge. It depends therefore on the employment of synthetical memory, and on the exercise of these higher functions of the cortex, which we have referred to when discussing apperception, concepts and reason. People vary enormously in the ability to use these functions, and the fundamental factor in this variability is probably innate. As has already been said, the newborn child possesses all the nerve cells he is going to have, but not all are able to function at once, because the nerve processes are not provided with their insulating myeline sheaths. These are only provided as further development takes place. Inasmuch as intelligence consists in the capacity for forming new groupings amongst the simpler engrams already laid down, the capacity for this function must depend in some measure on the number of neurones in the superficial layers of the cortex with which the individual is provided, since these cells subserve the highest function; and the age at which intelligence appears and develops will depend on the rate at which these cells acquire their myeline sheaths. Both of these factors are variants, and may account for the difference in individuals in this respect, for the study of the retarded personality reveals how the higher level structures of brains do differ. It is not easy to estimate the general intelligence of any personality, since the factor is essentially a complex integration of various capacities which depend very largely on environmental factors as to how they are displayed at any given time. Further consideration will be given to this subject in Chapter XV.

Of those personalities in whom new integrations of engrams arise to a greater extent than usual, with the result that original behaviour emerges, we say that they exhibit genius. This capacity for genius is generally admitted to be innate, but not to be identical with the possession of talents, which may be precocious but are essentially acquired. As we have seen, talents are examples of specially facilitated behaviour of a sort, which is familiar in the race, and which differs more in degree than in kind, from the pattern of behaviour exhibited by the average individual. Genius, on the other hand, is essentially the exhibition of a pattern of behaviour which is genuinely new, and differs in kind from the patterns exhibited by the rest of the community. The term "pattern of behaviour" is used in order to avoid narrowing the field of genius, since genius may be exhibited in manipulation, or in thought, in applied practical behaviour, or in abstract philosophical speculation. From this it is evident that the capacity to display a talent is innate, inasmuch as the engram concerned is innate; but the special facilitation which makes the engram subserve a talent, rather than an ordinary pattern of behaviour, is dependent on training and opportunity, though, in the more markedly precocious talents, this may be reduced to a minimum. To put it in another way, the disposition of the talented individual at birth does not materially differ from that of his less talented neighbour. On the other hand genius depends on an innate difference of disposition, namely the higher development of the superficial cortical neurones. None the less, it may require training and instruction to bring out the capacities of the genius. One other distinction is necessary to make. The talented man is frequently, if not always, a well-balanced individual, whereas a man of genius is only too often ill-balanced. The usual explanation, that genius requires for its appearance an agility and adaptability of mind which is impossible in the stable-minded, is only partially satisfying, and it would seem that we have to consider it from the aspect of different levels. The talented man is the highest example of a level which has "arrived" in the race, whereas the genius is a new departure, and new departures are never stable to begin with, but only achieve such stability after the function has become more generalized throughout the race. We may suggest therefore, that the products of contemporary genius become the talents of the future race, while contemporary talents become future instincts.

If talents, intelligence, and genius are functions of cortical integrations, involving cognition as the principal phase, there remains to consider the variation between individuals, dependent on the affective and conative integrations. It is clear that individuals will differ in the proportionate importance of the various emotional dispositions with which they are provided. Thus one person may have anger dominant and another fear. Under these circumstances, popular speech describes such people as being of an irascible disposition, or a timorous disposition, or again of an inquisitive disposition. However, in addition to this, McDougall has pointed out, that personalities vary in virtue of what he calls tempers, which are independent of the dominance of any particular impulse. He distinguishes three varieties of temper, (1) intensity or urgency, (2) persistency and (3) affectability. Acting on any impulse depending on a primary emotional disposition, a man may set out with a great energy and urgency, so that his activity is sudden and sharp, but this urgency may soon die down if the end is not immediately reached. Another may set out without such violence or speed, but may continue with the greatest persistency, until he has brought the activity to a successful conclusion. Again, a man may be easily affected by pleasure and unpleasure in his activity, so that he is much elated by success, and much cast down by failure. This is what McDougall calls affectability of temper, and this varies somewhat in its distribution. A man may be affected strongly both by pleasure and unpleasure, so that he is always very much up or very much down, or he may be very much affected by pleasure, but little affected by unpleasure, so that he is always buoyant and hopeful, or he may be much affected by unpleasure, but little by pleasure, so that he is always despondent. These differences are dependent on the organization of the engrams subserving the behaviour patterns and on the flow of activity through them. In the case of the urgent temper, the activation of any given engram is short and sharp and easily passes over to some other engraphic pattern. In the case of the persistent temper, the activation is slow, and the neuronic activity is maintained within the engram, passing on to other engrams with difficulty. In the temper characterized by affectability, the results of affective responses, involving, as they do, visceral and endocrine activity, easily modify the engraphic patterns, so that the correlated behaviour pattern is also changed. It is hard to explain how these modifications are brought about, unless it be by means of changes in the endocrine balance. Indeed, we know enough to recognize the affectability of the mild hyperthyroid individual, the persistency of the mild hyperpituitary, and the urgent activity of the mild hyperadrenal type. This indicates that the origin of the variation in tempers is to be sought in the temperamental factor, though our knowledge is not yet sufficiently exact to enable us to determine precisely the proportionate changes which are involved.

A similar explanation may be sought to account for moods. It has been said that the various endocrine secretions tend to intensify and perpetuate visceral nervous system activities. Thus it is known that certain physical changes, such as relaxation of the bronchioles, which are normally the result of sympathetic activity, may be intensified and perpetuated by keeping up an adequate supply of adrenalin in the circulating blood. Moods more or less correspond to emotions, and are referred to by similar names, such as angry, submissive, aggressive moods and the like. But they differ from emotions, inasmuch as they are more persistent as a rule, and are, to a certain extent, independent of emotions. Thus if I experience the emotion of anger, I am angry until that emotional reaction to a stimulus has passed, and some other stimulus with its appropriate emotional reactions intervenes, but if I am in an angry mood, I may experience some other stimulus to emotion while still in that mood, and to a certain extent react with the new emotion. I may be afraid or cheerful or anything else, though while I remain in an irritable mood, the emotion of anger is more easily aroused than if I am not in that mood. It would seem, then, that a mood is started by the corresponding emotion, but that it persists in the same way as the physical changes mentioned above persist, under the influence of adrenalin. We may conclude therefore, that the psychological statement that a mood is induced by emotion, but persists after the disappearance of the emotion, may be translated into physical terms as follows. An engram involving a special arrangement of vegetative neurones is activated, and under certain circumstances, varying with the individual and the nature of the stimulus, the corresponding pattern of endocrine activity is more than usually prominent, so that the period of activation of the neuronic engram is prolonged, and its irritability in the physiological sense is increased. Moody personalities are those whose endocrine system is specially susceptible to such activation.

In view of these variations between individual personalities, some of which are transitory and some of which are more or less permanent, many observers have attempted to classify the human race into groups, each characterized by some special type of personality. The recent work of the psycho-analytic schools has not only revived this study, but has given it a new orientation. This merits our further consideration, but before examining the doctrines of the various schools, it may be as well to consider how their views fit in with the standpoint adopted in this book. To begin with, we must recognize at once that their terminology, as usually expressed, is not in accordance with ours, and that if their doctrines are to be used or criticized, there must be a common ground of understanding as to terms. The most apparent inconsistency is in the use of the term libido. By libido, many of the psycho-analytic writers imply some special form of energy, whose origin and nature are by no means clear. Such an ill-defined conception we cannot admit, but, if we take a definition accepted by Jung, it may lead us back to a correlation with our point of view. The concept of energy is that which comes nearest to the concept of libido. Libido can perhaps be described as effect, or capacity for effect. It is capable of transformation from one form to another. The metamorphosis can be sudden, as when one function replaces another in a moment of danger, or it can be gradual, as we see it in that process of sublimation, where "the libido is led over a long and difficult path through a variety of forms into a different function". Our postulate has been that we have no right to presuppose any special form of energy acting within the body, other than that provided by the metabolism of the food, in a manner strictly analogous to the energy provided by the fuel in a combustion engine. We may put this in another way by saying that, with the emergence of life, the chief new function to be observed is the capacity for transforming potential energy into actual energy by a process we know as metabolism. Moreover the actual energy so liberated, may take the form of heat, chemical or electrical energy or of some other form, of whose nature we are ignorant, and which we are only capable of recognizing in the form of these other more familiar examples. So long as we recognize its common origin from the metabolized food, there is no particular objection to calling this energy libido, if it is convenient to do so. We may say then, that with the emergence of life, the body is capable of transforming the potential energy contained in the food, into the actual energy, libido, and, that by virtue of this energy, various integrated patterns of structures in the body are capable of activation and function. These patterns of structures are integrated and controlled through the function of the nervous system, so that one, when activated, subserves digestion, another locomotion, another circulation, and a fourth thought and so on. Hence we have no right to differentiate the energy or libido into thought libido, or digestive libido, or sex libido, or anything else, unless we are quite clear, that we are really talking of one and the same libido functioning in different ways, in virtue of the form of pattern of structures which is being activated at the moment. A good deal of confusion of thought is apt to arise, as a result of the failure to recognize such distinctions. For example, sex energy or sex libido is apt to be spoken of as if it was some terrific force, different from all other manifestations of energy in the body. It has been stated that, if the sex energy could only be harnessed to the function of thought, man would be capable of limitless intellectual achievement. If our contention is correct, sex energy is no different from thought energy, or digestive energy or any other energy. It is the same libido, the characteristic manifestation of the emergence of life, functioning in a special way, in virtue of the pattern which is in a state of activation. Yet there do seem to be differences between the "drive" of sex, and the "drive" of thought. Can such differences be explained? There seems no great difficulty. We have seen that the nervous system is essentially involved in all such patterns, that the synapses between the several neurones composing any given engram act as resistance boxes in the circuit which is being activated. Other things being equal therefore, the fewer synapses through which the activation has to pass, the more energy will be conserved, and the more "violent" will be the observed behaviour. Hence the simpler the pattern, and the lower the level in the nervous hierarchy, which is involved, the greater will be the "drive". But another factor comes in, that of inhibition and facilitation. By the former, resistance is increased to a maximum and the observable drive is diminished; by the latter, the resistance is reduced to a minimum, and the "drive" is increased. We should be more intelligible then, if, instead of talking about the transmutation of sex libido or sex energy into the function of thought, which would thereby increase the potentialities of man's intellect, we spoke of simplifying and facilitating the pattern subserving thought, so that it compared favourably with that of sex, in these respects. Then we might expect this increase in potentiality. Moreover, there are plenty of indications that by means of such short cuts, as language and capacity for form perception, this is actually taking place in the course of evolution, but we must not expect that by any process of psychic alchemy, man's capacities should change suddenly, any more than we can expect to change lead into gold by a simple chemical process. Having established this definition of the libido, as a characteristic manifestation of life, we may allow that in the course of evolution the organization of structural patterns has been so constituted, that the emergent behaviour patterns differ considerably, and the general "go" of the personality is oriented in various directions. With the emergence of life two functions must be fulfilled, the preservation of the race and the preservation of the individual. Moreover, if we examine the constitution of the individual at a low level, before matters have become too complicated, we may recognize, that certain of his dispositions function chiefly to serve self-preservation, and others to serve race-preservation. Thus at the level of the appetities, it is clear that the nutritive appetites subserve the function of self-preservation, while that of sex subserves the preservation of the race. Primitive fear and anger are chiefly concerned with the individual, but may be so organized as to function in respect of race. Conversely, primitive sympathy and negativity are primarily concerned with race-preservation, but may under certain circumstances be organized in the service of the individual. Some authorities put gregariousness as a function comparable to race- and self-preservation, but this would seem to be erroneous, for gregariousness is not universal like the other two, and is a more complicated organization, emerging at a higher level, and at a later stage in evolutionary progress.

If we examine the biographies of individuals we find that one person is so organized that the whole trend of his behaviour is directed towards the preservation of the individual, and the conservation of his interests. Another person, on the contrary, shows by his behaviour that his organization is towards race- preservation and conservation of its interests. It is clear, of course, that no individual can entirely rid himself of the concerns of the race, or of the ego respectively; but the organization towards race-preservation behaviour, or sex, in the one, is more facilitated, while the reverse is the case in the other. It is clear that behaviour concerned with the race is directed away from the ego, and is therefore objective, while behaviour concerned with the individual is directed towards the ego, and is subjective. The psycho-analysts talk of one individual as displaying centrifugal, or sex libido, while the other displays centripetal, or ego libido. We have seen that such use of the word libido, is only permissible under the most strict reservations, and on the understanding that we are really talking of a facilitation of a special structural organization, rather than of the flow of a special form of energy.

Freud, the founder of psycho-analysis, was an empiricist and one of the most acute clinical observers in medical history. He therefore naturally turned his attention to the sex, or objective aspect, in the biography of his patients. Like many others of his type, his observations were often more valuable than the conclusions he drew from them, and consequently his insistence that the objective sex libido determines everything, does not find acceptance as a true philosophical explanation, as opposed to a convenient hypothesis, unless it be with the relatively few, who are content to accept a convenient hypothesis as truth, and to whom, by reason of other personal characteristics, into whose nature we need not enter here, this particular hypothesis proves acceptable. It is clear that early in the history of the movement, some who were interested in the subjective aspect, would turn their attention to the subjective organization in the biographies under observation. As it happened, a brilliant disciple of Freud, of a more than usually subjective type, was found in the person of Adler, and he naturally turned his attention to the "ego-libido," and sought to explain things in terms of this, as exclusively, as Freud sought to use "sex libido." Obviously between the extreme objective view and the extreme subjective view, there could be no compromise and indeed the antagonism was bitter. This however, is useful from our point of view, for by studying Freud we gain insight into the individual organized in respect of centrifugal race-preservation behaviour, and by studying Adler we gain insight into the individual organized in respect of centripetal self-preservation behaviour.

There still remains however, another serious split in the psycho-analytic school, which was as inevitable as the other. In our study of the instincts we had occasion to notice the close connexion between the sex and constructive instincts, and suggested that they might be regarded as branches from one tree. Further, we drew attention to the fact, that in man they had been largely diverted from their original biological purpose, and harnessed to serve his own satisfaction and pleasure. These satisfactions may be sought in the purely objective world of reality, by always pursuing objects outside the ego, or the individual may pursue these satisfactions in the more subjective realm of phantasy, the realm of prospective imagination, of dreams, of art and creative genius. So here again, we have a cleavage in the race of those who are organized towards sex- and race-preservation, between those who are integrated purely objectively towards sex, in the more usually accepted sense of the term, and those who are organized towards creation and prospective imagination. So, in the individual personality, there is a similar cleavage; for, as has been said, no individual is simple, though one or other organization is more facilitated and constitutes a more definite and clearly marked engram. As might be expected, this led to a further development in psycho-analytic research. Freud, the extreme objectivist, ruthlessly pursued the objective organization of sex, while the subjectivist Jung fixed his interests on the realm of phantasy and creation, and studied this type in the race, and this organization in the individual. This may be represented diagrammatically as follows:—

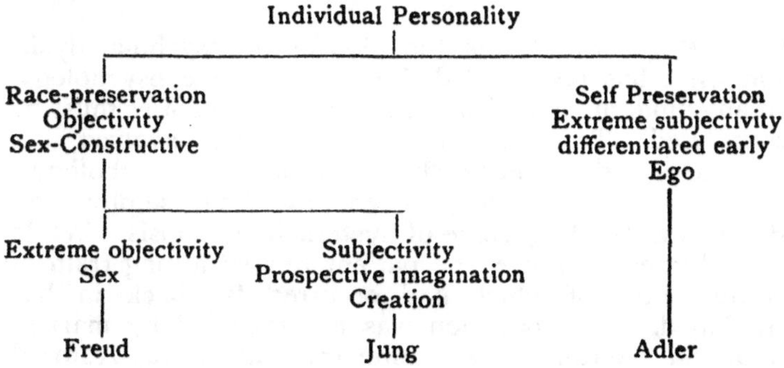

From this, we may see, how a critical study of these three observers who have turned their attention specifically to the three aspects of personality, may be of great service to a proper conception of the whole. To such we may now turn our attention.

CHAPTER IX

THE CONTRIBUTION OF FREUD TO THE STUDY OF PERSONALITY

SIGMUND FREUD[1] was the pioneer of psycho-analysis, and what has been called the new dynamic psychology. In any modern psychological study, these theories must be considered. To understand clearly what is involved, it is necessary to describe briefly how this new "psychology" came into being. In the year 1880, the Viennese physician Breuer was treating a case of hysteria by hypnosis. While in an hypnotic trance, the patient related a long train of events, some of which had occurred far back in her childhood. The narration was accompanied by marked emotional excitement, and after the patient was restored to full consciousness, her general condition was considerably improved. Following the suggestion offered on this occasion, Breuer and Freud investigated the effect of what they called abreaction. This they describe as the freeing of "confined affect," which occurs when the patient is induced to relate an experience which was originally accompanied by considerable affective reaction, and which has not been allowed to come into consciousness for some considerable time. What really happens is that the engram, which subserves the set of ideas relating to the experience, is reassociated, so that it achieves that relatedness which involves consciousness. So, from the psychological aspect, the experience is reintegrated with proper relation to time and space, and in proper proportion to the rest of the personality. It is this reintegration which induces the therapeutic benefit, and not the mere ebullition of emotional excitement. This relief by "abreaction" is familiar in present-day psychotherapy, but its investigators soon found that abreaction in itself was not enough, in many cases of neurosis. Freud thereupon turned his attention away from pure therapeutics, and initiated an enquiry into the mental processes of neurotics. Even so recently as 1920 he remarks, "At the present time theoretical knowledge is still far more important to all of us than therapeutic success."

This enquiry into the neurotic mind was strictly empirical, and Freud deliberately turned his back on a priori suppositions derived from the orthodox psychology of the time. As a result of his studies, he formulated a new conception of psychological processes, or rather expressed what was partly old in a different way. In common with most psychologists, he recognized that the individual started life with certain hereditary dispositions, and he was content to group these broadly into two divisions, Ego and Sex. He laid stress however on the "structure" of these dispositions, and pointed out that a conation or wish is involved, leading the individual to strive for its gratification, and this demand for gratification he termed the pleasure principle. In other words he contended that there is a "set," inherent in the nature of these dispositions, which makes for that immediate satisfaction in the relief of tension which is termed pleasure. He further recognized that at a very early stage in the life of a child, the set of his dispositions towards pleasure is opposed by the influence of environment. This latter he termed the reality principle, which would seem to correspond to certain aspects of what Trotter[2] calls the herd instinct, but which would be better described as the community attitude. Freud refers to the dread of society as a potent factor in modifying the activity of the basal complexes, and this is indeed the chief influence to act upon the primary dispositions. It is obvious that conflict must arise between these two principles in every individual, and Freud maintained that the origin of the psychoneuroses depended on the failure to find an adequate solution of this conflict, and the establishment of a compromise which was not a satisfactory adaptation to circumstances. Continuing his investigations in the light of his own interests, as explained in the last chapter, he was led to the conclusion that the vast majority, if not all cases of psychoneuroses, depended on a failure in adaptation between the pleasure principle associated with sex, and the reality principle. More recently, he has somewhat modified this standpoint, and admitted the influence of other dispositions in the production of neuroses. As he pointed out, it was not unlikely to be true that sex, in the narrow sense, played the dominant part in conflict with reality, inasmuch as a child is usually trained in the adaptation of his other impulses to environmental requirements from the very first, whereas little or no effort is made to teach him, or help him, to adapt his sex impulse. But in Freud's use of the term sex complex, he includes much more than the impulse to direct sexual gratification, applying the term to the complete sentiment we call love. As a result of his studies of the mind of children, and his investigations into the apparently forgotten memories of adults, Freud was convinced that manifestations of the sexual impulse were present at a very much earlier stage, than was usually regarded as probable, and that these exerted an influence of paramount importance on the future psychic development of the individual. He attributes to sex, therefore, a much greater importance in the shaping of a personality than we have indicated in the previous chapters. Most of his critics accept the general principles of conflict, and recognize its influence in distinguishing between various personalities, and in preventing that harmonious development which is desirable, but seldom, if ever, achieved. They consider, however, that he and his followers have insisted too much on the universality of the sex impulse as the protagonist against reality, and have thought that the egocentric impulses may also determine difficulties. But as has been said, this has been to a certain extent admitted by Freud in his later works. Also, they criticize the view of Freud, that any early pleasurable feeling, such as is exhibited in feeding at the breast, is necessarily sexual feeling. This however may be more a difference in the use of terms than a fundamental disagreement, for Freud maintains that any effort to attain contact with an object in the environment is sexual, while the critics, who have refused to accept his conclusions with regard to the actual sexuality of many of his interpretations of childish impulses, would not admit such a wide connotation of the word sexual. Its use, moreover, is misleading and, as Bernard Hart puts it, a legitimate criticism of the psychoanalytic school may be illustrated by the following analogy. Suppose an inhabitant from another planet were placed outside a room, and told to form his opinion of the inhabitants of this world by his observations of the people who came out of this room. The inmates were then all passed through a mangle, so that they were rolled out flat, before they issued from it. The inference would be that the inhabitants of this world were all two-dimensional. Is it not possible that psycho-analysis, in the strict sense of the term, works somewhat as that mangle works, and makes the mental processes of every person, who is subjected to it, appear to be sexually determined? This question, however, of the universality of sexual influence in the conflict between the individual and his environment, need not detain us here, for most people will be agreed, that the real value of Freud's work does not involve an insistence on this universality. It must be admitted, however, by any honest critic, that at any rate so far as psychoneurotics are concerned, and so far as the behaviour of a great many normal people is concerned, sexual impulses and their maladaptations to reality do have an enormous influence in shaping their behaviour. Freudians would probably say that this denial of sexuality in all conflict is the attitude of the prejudiced man who is unwilling to admit the truth of a new doctrine, established by scientific enquiry. But this attitude is by no means unhealthy, and is certainly to be preferred to that which embraces new theories, and presumes they are facts, before sufficient evidence has been collected to support them.

To return to Freud's teaching with regard to the conflict between the individual dispositions, and the environment or reality, which is of first-class importance in the study of Personality, he pointed out that the ideal outcome of such a conflict is that some adaptation between them should be achieved. In this way, a working compromise is obtained, which will allow the individual to live in his environment with a minimum of friction. We may say without prejudice, that at the present stage of evolution at any rate, a completely frictionless adaptation is never achieved, and it is this fact which makes Freud's work valuable in the study of so-called normal individuals, as well as in the realm of psychopathology. When, in the case of conflict, friction becomes too great, the only possible solutions are by the establishment of logic-tight compartments, or by what is called repression. By the former is meant a more or less conscious refusal to let the two conflicting complexes be considered together, and it is only possible, when the conflicting complexes do not deeply involve the affective organizations of the personality. Again, in the mind of the child, or the primitive, in whom the power of logical reasoning has not yet developed, logic-tight compartments may exist, simply through failure of integration. Many of the religious beliefs of primitive, and even of civilized people, are logically quite incompatible, and yet are held in consciousness without any conflict. By repression is meant that since the individual actually cannot get rid of reality, or of his disposition, he must do his best to persuade himself that the experience or the disposition, which are incompatible with each other, no longer exist. As, for example, when sex impulse is misdirected, many people persuade themselves that they possess no sex feeling at all. Such rejected material becomes unconscious, and may cease to develop with the rest of the personality. Repressed material may consist of dispositions which have never functioned, or of acquired experience which is incompatible. As Freud himself expresses it "Man's archaic heritage forms the nucleus of the unconscious mind, and whatever part of that heritage has to be left behind in the advance to later phases of development, because it is useless, or incompatible with what is new, and harmful to it, falls a victim to the process of repression." The same is true of acquired experiences which cannot be adapted to reality. The individual cannot completely divorce such a disposition or experience from his personality, but he can and does divorce it, so far as consciousness is concerned; or, in other words, the engram which subserves it, from whichever aspect we care to regard it, ceases to enjoy that relatedness which involves consciousness. The subject, so to speak, turns his back on this trait in his character, or experience of his environment, and refuses to recognize that it is there, and by means of this process of repression actually ceases to believe in its existence. It is no longer integrated so as to be orientated in time and space, and indeed becomes dissociated from the rest of conscious material. It is only such material, which has thus been repressed, which becomes a complex in the strict Freudian sense of the term, just as an unrepressed set of ideas, accompanied by affect, is termed a constellation. Repression may be more or less successful. If the repressed complex is one which seldom comes into opposition with the world of reality in which the individual lives, or with his dispositions as the case may be—so that it represents but an unimportant element in the personality—he may go through life without any disturbance, and repression is successful. In this sense repression is a useful function which is constantly in evidence throughout life. This success however, is not always achieved, and repression may be incompletely successful, or even entirely unsuccessful. In the latter case, normal existence in the face of an unresolved complex is impossible, and the individual either becomes neurotic, or may even find a solution in suicide.

To allow the continuance of existence in relation to the environment to go on, the repressed complex, and all images or instances in the past which are closely associated with it, and which tend to become stimuli which reactivate the engram subserving it, must be kept below the level of the active consciousness of the individual. This state of affairs is achieved by what Freud terms the censor. This we may examine, although the somewhat anthropomorphic conceptions tend to obscure clear thinking.

For the purpose of this concept he divides the mind into three territories, sometimes described as layers of consciousness. The difference between these territories lies in their special degree and manner of relatedness, and mental processes may pass from one to the other in gaining or losing that relatedness, which subserves their existence in one or other territory or layer. The highest he calls the "conscious," wherein all mental processes of which the individual is aware have their being, that is, those processes are in consciousness which enjoy that relatedness involving reflective thought. Below this, is the layer of the fore-conscious, where all mental processes exist of which the subject is not aware at any moment, but which can easily be brought to mind. There is a more or less continuous interchange of mental processes from the fore-conscious to the conscious layer, because there is no marked difficulty for the processes in the fore-conscious achieving that relatedness which involves consciousness. It may be, however, that some groups of ideas less easily become fully conscious than others. This inhibition of complete integration is what Freud calls the censor. Thus, a weak censorship may be said to exist between conscious and fore-conscious, but it is one which is easily overcome, and which does not exert any marked influence on the mental life of the subject. The third layer is termed by Freud the unconscious, and in this, these mental processes have their being which under no ordinary circumstances can be brought into consciousness. Some of these complexes may never have been conscious, others may have been conscious at one time, but have been repressed, so that they are not recalled. According to the Freudians, this prohibition is exercised by the censor, whose business it is to refuse admission to consciousness of any complex which is strongly imbued with unpleasant affect and, if we regard the censor as a process of inhibition, we have already remarked on the influence of unpleasant affect in establishing inhibition. The mental material found to be unconscious will be those hereditary dispositions which have not been adjusted to the reality of the environment, and also the images of the unpleasant incidents which have been responsible for the acute conflicts of these dispositions with reality. It will thus be seen, that part of the "content of the unconscious" is "material" derived from the hereditary dispositions, and part is "material" derived from acquired experience, and that all this "material" is unconscious, because of failure in adaptation to reality. This aspect of inhibition at psychological levels is analogous to that at physiological levels, and just as antagonist muscles must be inhibited so that agonists may function, so "antagonist" complexes must be inhibited, in order that the rest of the personality may function.

As was said above, success of the censor in maintaining the repression of these complexes depends on their importance, relative to the rest of the personality, and the frequency with which they are stimulated into activity by the environment. If the repression is completely successful the complexes are pragmatically non-existent, because they never influence conscious thought or behaviour, under any circumstances. If, however, repression is not completely successful, the complexes so far as the individual awareness is concerned are forgotten, but will influence behaviour in some way or other. The analogy so commonly drawn, between the Freudian censorship and the censor of a country at war, is an excellent one. Enemy subjects within the country cannot get information outside by direct means, but may be able to do so, by means of subterfuges and codes which cheat the censor, and hence escape his vigilance. Freud contends that these unconscious complexes may find expression, or partial expression, in consciousness in symbolic form, and that the explanation of certain otherwise inexplicable factors in human behaviour depends on the recognition of this symbolical expression of repressed complexes. In other words, inhibition may be incomplete, and though activation of the engram, subserving the image of the original experience, may be impossible, activation may spread to associated engrams, which subserve symbolic representations of that experience. Examples of such behaviour have been worked out, and are described at length in the literature of psycho-analysis, in the cases of dreams, reveries, certain artistic expressions, personal mannerisms and eccentricities, slips of the tongue and slips of the pen, and many other everyday occurrences. The criticisms of these explanations of Freud are that he implies some sort of drive or impulsion, which so to speak forces out the symbolic abnormal thought or behaviour, whereas such thought or behaviour may more properly be regarded as a new emergent from eccentric combinations of impulses, depending on inhibitions and facilitations. These latter may be determined by processes and reactions such as are described by Freud.

Other conceptions of the Freudian psychology which demand particular notice, are the wish and the libido. For Freud and his "dynamic" psychology, the unit of mental process is the wish. This is the "setting" of an engram towards some active conation, which is consequent on the stimulus of an object or objects in the environment. This "wish" may be appetitive or aversive. As Holt[3] has pointed out, this treatment of the wish, as the important phase for examination, is new in psychology, and of the greatest value. The principal attribute of living, as opposed to dead protoplasm, is that living matter reacts to its environment. That is to say, that a new factor comes into existence with that relatedness we call life, namely, that a living organism can receive impressions from its environment, and by its own activity modify its environment. The first may to a certain extent be true of dead matter, for it may receive impressions from its environment, in the shape of a blow or any other application of force; but it cannot be said to modify its environment by reason of its own activity, except in such a circumscribed and more or less constant fashion as is observed in radioactivity. This conception of modification of the environment demands an accompanying concept of activity, in relationship to the environment, but it is by no means necessary to imply that there is a conscious end in view in this related activity. When an amœba flows towards a food particle and ingests it, there is certainly an activity in relationship to the food particle, which involves a certain purpose, namely assimilation of food, but we may be certain that there is no such conscious end in view, as is described by some as an "act of will." This purposive mental process, with relation to the environment, is the Freudian wish, and so far as can be judged from Freud's own works, he means no more than this. However, the writings of some of his followers imply a great deal more, and suggest a consciously purposeful process or "act of will." This is certainly misleading. Freud, then, would postulate that his unconscious complexes involve wishes, that is to say that they have from their very organization, a purposive relation to their environment, which, allowed to develop, will modify the latter in some way. He would imply however, in opposition to Adler, as will be seen later, that the striving towards an object is determined and organized by the constitution of the dispositions, and not from the constitution of the end in view. The modification of the environment is the objective aspect of such a wish. There is also a subjective aspect, which for want of a better term we may call a gratification of the wish. This is, after all, identical with the relief of tension, which constitutes pleasure. Freud, as has been said, declares that the unconscious complexes, by virtue of their very structural nature, are alway striving for gratification, and that the reality principle stands in their way. This conflict is followed by repression, symbolical representations and the rest. This conception of striving for gratification necessitates the concept of some sort of energy, which he calls libido. This has been discussed in the last chapter, and as has been seen, the Freudian statement cannot be accepted without modification. Subject to this however, we may describe libido as the form of energy, whatever its nature may be, which enables the wish to become translated into active behaviour. In the process of growth, the wishes as they come into contact with the reality principle are more or less successfully integrated and modified, and by this integration, the individual reaches a higher level in the hierarchy of behaviour. At first they are entirely egocentric, or, to use Janet's[4] expression, their radius of action is confined to one individual. Later they become integrated on to higher and higher levels, and their radius of action, expands *pari passu* with their development, so that the behaviour which results from the integration of these wishes becomes more and more complicated. If the development is successful, and repressions do not occur, or are successful by the process of normal fusion and suppression, to use Rivers's terms, then the original egocentric wishes become changed into more socially desirable impulses. This modification is what Freud means by the term sublimation. By this process of sublimation the constitution of the complexes is so changed, that the wishes involved work towards a different and more desirable end.

No individual at any period of his life stands still, and with the continual development of the personality, old stages in the growth of that personality are left behind, and old types of reaction are discarded. They are not however incapable of revival, for if, at any time, the difficulty of adaptation between the reality principle and the growing personality becomes too great, regression may occur. By regression we mean that there is a harking back to previous levels of development, so that, for example, the adult may go back to childish behaviour. This process of regression is an everyday experience, both in normal and pathological conditions. It is within the experience of every family, and of every married couple, that when one member does not get what he wants, he or she is apt to regress, and behave like a child, may even talk baby language, and perform some old childish tricks which have been long left behind, so far as everyday use is concerned; but, as a rule, these processes are temporary, and the individual quickly regains touch with reality, and proceeds with his personal development and adaptation. When however, the conflict is too severe, it may happen that the regression is much more serious, and the individual goes back more permanently to a childish type of behaviour. Since he finds this will not work in the environment in which he is, he has by force of circumstances, to try and make a new environment. This he may do, by withdrawing from reality as it surrounds him, and refusing to admit that it is such as it is. Instead, he weaves for himself a new environment of phantasy, in which he loses himself. Such a state of affairs is seen in its extreme degree in certain cases of dementia præcox, but we are all apt to take refuge from the hard facts of real existence by building for ourselves castles in the air. Regression, then, is a direct consequence of conflict, and is a method, albeit unsatisfactory, of compromising with reality.

A further corollary to the process of conflict and repression is the active process of forgetting, and Freud offers a full explanation of this. It is part of the general doctrine of repression, that experiences of incidents which are disagreeable to the individual, that is to say, charged with unpleasant affective tone, tend to be relegated to "the unconscious" and kept there by "the censor," and the degree to which they are repressed, and the success of the censorship, will depend on the intensity of this unpleasant tone in relation to the ego. That this is a common mode of forgetting, scarcely anyone will deny. We do tend to forget all sorts of things, which are in opposition to our amour-propre, and it is these things which are most unpleasant to the ego. We do not tend so much to forget things which have simply interfered with the normal activities or development of our personalities, if we have no particular ideal in phantasy connected with this activity. But, whenever there is a sense of shame, or remorse, or a feeling that we are failing to come up to the ideal we set ourselves, the incidents concerned are very readily put out of mind. Whenever there is an arraignment of ourselves before the judgment-seat of our ego, then intense painful affect is experienced, and the incident which is responsible for this state of affairs tends to be repressed. The Freudians suggest that the whole of the amnesia of infantile experience, that is to say, of experiences before the age of five, which are forgotten, are repressed in this way, because they are not compatible with ideals established as the infant grows to childhood, and that memory of these experiences can be restored by special methods. The chief of these methods is psycho-analysis. This is a difficult statement on which to deliver a fair judgment, for the obvious criticism is, that the psycho-analyst has a preconceived idea of what he will find, and suggests this to the patient, who produces for his gratification various aspects of the so-called Œdipus complex. The reply of the psycho-analysts is that suggestion is never used, and that similarities in the working of the infantile mind are biologically probable, just as are similarities of the infantile body, which are much closer to the norm than are the bodies of adults. Further, they claim the pragmatic sanction, since they maintain, that restoration of these infantile memories removes neurotic symptoms. This, they contend, would not ensue unless the memories were true representations of personal incidents. Their explanation is that the activities of the child at that time, represent crude gratifications of wishes, mostly connected with the sexual impulse, which later become impossible when brought up against reality; and with the growth of the individual, and his adaptations to reality, it becomes intolerable that he should have ever carried out, or wished to carry out, such behaviour. To many people the claim that in all instances of forgetting this explanation is applicable, seems to be going too far, and as Professor Pear[6] pointed out, it seems more rational to account for forgetting at this age, and later in life, under three heads. Firstly, incidents are forgotten when they have not made sufficient impression on the individual, either because of their unimportance, or because of their insufficient distinctiveness from the general course of ideas of the subject. For example, we do not remember the number of the railway carriage in which we travelled three years ago, because this was not sufficiently important to make any impression upon our consciousness, and so far as observation carries us, this memory is completely lost, and cannot be restored by the utmost exploration of the unconscious mind, whether in the waking or in the hypnotic state. The second subgrouping in this category may be illustrated by conversation in a political club, when all the members think alike. In such a case, the remarks of each one correspond too closely to the trend of thought of any member to be clearly recollected. However, let a person of opposite political convictions come in and join in an argument, and his remarks will be clearly remembered. The second head under which forgetting may be dealt with, is the Freudian one of repression, that is to say, the refusal to tolerate the ideas charged with unpleasant feeling tone in consciousness. The third head, with which he deals, he describes under the name supersession. By this, he means that the individual is continually changing and continually growing. Hence certain groups of ideas are superseded by others, and the earlier group is left behind, and no longer comes to consciousness. To what extent this group is really differentiated from the group of repression is doubtful, because, as Freud said, it is the earlier constellations which are no longer useful, or which are painful to the individual, which come to be repressed, and Professor Pear's superseded group would seem to be those constellations which are no longer useful to the individual. This third group is therefore only a subdivision of repression.

So far reference has been made to the aspects of Freudian Psychology in relation to the mental activities of everyday life, but one cannot adequately deal with these without mentioning his work in connexion with the symptoms of the neuroses. Many people will consider that once we embark on this line of enquiry we are necessarily stepping from the normal into the pathological; but an error, which many psychologists have made in the past, has been that they have regarded the average mind as much too well balanced, and much too tidy. It was this error that made psychology so little use for medical purposes at the time when Freud began his investigations. This mistake is due to the fact that the majority of academic psychologists, who work by introspection, are of the type described by James as tender-minded. Such people have a horror of loose ideas, and their notions, as a rule, are arranged in careful logical sequence. They do not allow their thoughts to wander in an inconsequent way. The description, therefore, which they deduce from the observations of their own mental processes is bound to represent the logical and well-ordered mind. For this reason, the text-books of many psychologists entirely neglect the extreme incoherence of the minds of many people, and only describe the mental processes of one class of individuals. The neurotic might be described as an individual with an abnormally untidy mind. In such cases the instabilities, illogicalities of the average man, obtrude themselves in an obvious and unmistakable way. Further, a study of the symptoms complained of by these neurotics does not necessarily mean an excursion into pathological psychology, but, on the contrary, may throw a flood of light on the personality of the average man. It is a characteristic of the psychoneurotic, as opposed to those who are insane, that however unsuccessfully, he is making an effort to adapt to circumstances, and even the most normal man has to struggle continually to adapt himself.

For Freud, the psychoneuroses depend on a failure of adaptation between the sexual impulses and the reality principle, and the various symptoms of the neuroses are symbolical representations of sexual wishes which have been denied gratification by the reality principle, or of unsatisfactory compromises arrived at in the struggle. Since this conflict between sex and reality involves painful affect, the wishes have been more or less repressed. Repression in these cases is not successful, and the censor is not strong enough to keep all manifestations of these ungratified wishes out of consciousness. According to Freud, the gross hysterical symptoms such as paralysis, blindness, sensory changes, and the like, are physical expressions of this wish, and may be regarded as crystallized protests against their non-gratification. From this, he concludes that, in order to cure an hysterical symptom, it is necessary to find the repressed wish, and enable the individual to avoid repression, by discovering a method of gratification, other than that forbidden by reality. This new gratification may be found in higher and more adult developments of the primitive or childish wish. Such process of outlet along higher channels has already been referred to as sublimation. The pathogenesis of hysterical symptoms does not concern us here, but the process of sublimation, is of great importance. Whereas, at the developmental level of the primitive or the child, a wish may only be gratified in a primitive physical way, at the adult level, the same wish may have been so altered by the processes of development and supersession that it finds its gratification through affective and intellectual channels. Sublimation is the basis of many social and conventional practices. For example, collecting is a sublimation of the acquisitive impulse, restrained and controlled, according to the dictates of the community, while dancing is to some extent a sublimation of the sex impulse and so on. Moreover, sublimations involve a great degree of integration and control, and hence are of considerable educative value. For instance, although other factors are involved, real climbing and other dangerous sports are in some sense a sublimation of the fear-flight impulse, and they certainly involve an education in the control of fear, which may be of great use to the individual. Hence this process of sublimation is the method by which the reactions of the personality grow and evolve under the influence of experience and education. In the case of the hysteric, certain reactions are dissociated and left behind, in the process of general growth, and in order to remove symptoms these reactions have to be sublimated, or brought into line with the rest of the personality. In the normal, all reactions do not grow at equal rates, and hence in every one of us sublimation is necessary in one way or another.

Turning to another form of psychoneuroses, the Freudians regard the affective manifestations of anxiety hysteria to be due to the failure to gratify primitive sexual wishes, either directly, or by way of sublimation. Such manifestations as phobias, manias, etc., are symbolic objective fixations, which take the place of the real fixation, which is sexual, and the unpleasant affective tone, consequent in failure to achieve gratification of the wish, achieves a new fixation. The word fixation is used to describe the "set" of the individual towards, or away from, some object in the environment. For example, a patient suffering from a "mania" may be unable to avoid the impulse to wash his hands frequently, while one with a phobia may be unable to bring himself to cross a street. The washing of hands is usually a symbolical effort to cleanse himself of guilt, and the affect really appertaining to the real or imagined guilt is attached to the relatively unimportant idea of soiled hands. Similarly, the dread of a phobia, really applies to fear least some guilty (generally sexual) deed be performed, but becomes secondarily attached, or fixed, to an apparently harmless act, such as crossing a street. Such extreme fixations are not met with in the normal person, yet which of us have not got some irrational attraction or repulsion for certain objects, which to others seem quite indifferent. The explanation of such attitudes may be found to lie in the fact that the objects, though having little value in themselves, are symbolic of other objects, of great value to the personality, whether according to adult standards, or more often, according to childish standards.

The field in which Freudian psychology, in connexion with the neuroses, has attracted most attention is undoubtedly the interpretation of dreams. It has been a belief, all through the history of mankind, that dreams do mean something, and that they can be interpreted. From Joseph and Daniel to Old Moore, dream interpreters have been found. Freud, however, was the first to invest such interpretations with a scientific spirit, and to give an explanation of the mechanism of dreams. With the materialistic wave of the 19th century, dreams were regarded as too fantastic to be worthy of the notice of the true scientist, and they were dismissed as being due to such physical causes as lying on the back, eating indigestible things at supper, or changes in the blood pressure. Although these explanations may determine the occurrences of dreams—that is to say, they may make sleep sufficiently light to allow the dreamer to be aware, both that he is dreaming, and that he is dreaming about some definite thing—they do nothing to explain the cognitive and affective contents of dreams. Freud's theory is that the dream is an expression of unconscious wishes, just as neurotic symptoms are, though he would admit that in certain simple dreams, and in the common dreams of children, these wishes are by no means necessarily unconscious. A child who has been forbidden sweets during the daytime, will dream of eating them at night; but that does not mean the wish for sweets has been at any time unconscious in the Freudian sense of the term. In the neurotic however, Freud holds that the same wishes, which are giving rise to the symptoms of the patient, will find partial expression in the dreams of that patient, but it will only be very rarely that the expression will be direct. The censor, though relatively relaxed, is still active during sleep, and the wish has to take on a symbolic form. Freud explains the readiness with which dreams are forgotten, by the fact that when the patient awakens, the censor again becomes fully active and reimposes full repression on the complex. Furthermore, there is no proper integration of the various wishes which constitute the mental content during sleep. Hence, many diverse wishes, connected with diverse complexes, may find expression in the same dream. Diverse sets of ideas and images may be superimposed on each other, so as to give an almost unidentifiable picture, analogous to a composite photograph, such as Galton delighted in; but, when unravelled and explained, they are found to be expressions of these unconscious repressed complexes, which are disturbing the peaceful integration of the personality. The study of dreams serves to show the importance of the wish in psychology, and how an activation once started, may spread through all sorts of unexpected engraphic paths. It illustrates how complicated are the neuronic arrangements at the highest levels, yet how, with patient study, these patterns may be unravelled, and the process of integration understood. The processes whereby dreams or other symbolic representations, such as neurotic symptoms, may be investigated and determined, comprise the art of psycho-analysis.

The object of this art is to discover the imperfectly repressed complexes, and disentangle them from the resistances which are established under the censor, and which prevent the gratification of the wishes which determine them. The chief method of psycho-analysis is free association. The patient is encouraged to let his stream of consciousness flow without any attempt at purposeful guidance, and in this way symbolic representations are frequently reattached to their original meaning, and the experienced physician may recognize, firstly in what directions the resistances lie, and secondly what repressed material these resistances cover. When studying dreams by this process, it is found that the contents of a dream, however nonsensical it may appear, are definitely determined, and that certain laws apply to the formation of dream contents and serve to explain the images which appear in it, and their arrangements one to another. Freud has laid stress on the affect in dreams, and emotional association is often a valuable means of establishing relationships between the symbol and the original. By this latter expression is meant a recollection of a situation, in which a similar emotion to that felt in the dream was experienced. The methods of interpreting dreams are fully described in psycho-analytic literature, and are of interest in the study of personality, inasmuch as they illustrate the presence and influence of repressed complexes, even in non-pathological cases. A dream is always associated with the ego, and if, as sometimes is the case, the dreamer does not seem to come into the picture at all, it is fairly certain that he is there under some disguise or other. For this reason also, dream investigation may be of considerable use in the study of personality. Freud regards the function of the dream as being bivalent. It is partly a means of outlet for repressed material. However, if this strongly effective material were to become conscious without adequate disguise, the subject would awake, as happens in nightmares. Hence the various disguises and symbolizations instituted by the "censor," keeps the subject asleep by preventing too strongly affective material from entering consciousness. He maintains that the dream is always the fulfilment of some sort of wish, though this wish may be a negative wish, that is to say, a desire for avoidance, as opposed to a positive wish, or desire for fulfilment or appetition. That this is a commonly accepted explanation of dreams is made obvious from many illustrations in literature, but it may suffice to recall the remark of Plato, "That a good man dreams what a bad man does." Freud considers that dreams always have a relation to past tendencies in the individual, that is to say, tendencies which existed in childhood, and have persisted in a repressed form till the present day, and that these tendencies are sexual in nature. Jung on the other hand, thinks that this is too indiscriminate, that great care should always be taken to be quite sure that what is termed a sexual symbol is necessarily so for the patient. This might be illustrated by the following dream. An ex-soldier dreamt of being very terrified by the presence of a large snake on his shoulders. A snake is a well known sexual symbol, and the Freudians would probably say the dream referred to some sexual complex, and would no doubt find one by going right back into the childhood of the patient. His associations with this dream, however, had reference to his most terrifying experience during the war. When on guard outside a camp, and standing under a wall, a large snake had slithered down over the wall and over his shoulder. This dream had been persistent, but disappeared when a connexion was established with this incident; and it is difficult to see why one should have to go right back to childhood to find some sexual explanation of such a dream, when the more obvious explanation served to remove it. Jung considers that a dream has a good deal to do with the patient's tendencies in the present, and may have significance in relation to what the patient is going to do. He regards dreams as being a useful guidance as to the progress of the patient, and considers that when the patient dreams of things in closer relation to the practical work of the world, that this is a good sign. For Jung, then, the dream may be teleological, and is a symbolic picture of the subconscious strivings of the patient's wakening life. This view held by Jung is valuable, but must not be carried too far, as once any psychological process is looked upon as prophetic, there is no limit to the flight of speculative ideas which may be deduced from this concept. With regard to simple symbolism in dreams, an example may make clear what is meant. A boy who had been very troubled with war nightmares, which are of course direct representations of repressed or partially repressed complexes, was getting better, and adapting himself more successfully to the prospects of the future, and his reflections as to his behaviour in the past. However, that he was not free from his repression was shown by the fact that he had the following dream. He was in a billiard room, and was playing at the red ball, aiming at a pocket, and had a feeling that if he did not get it down into the pocket something dreadful would happen. Taking the incidents of the dream seriatim, the billiard room proved a simple wish fulfilment, comparable to the childish dream, as it represented the place where he spent most of his spare time at home. His immediate association with a red ball was a bursting shell, and of that with getting it down into the pocket, the absolute necessity of getting away from it, down a dug-out. This dream enabled us to restore an amnesia which previously had not been discovered. He had given the history that he had known nothing from the time when he was in a trench, to the time when he reached the dressing station. Now however, he remembered that he had been at the top of the dug-out steps with his sergeant, that a shell had burst close to them, which killed the sergeant, and knocked him all the way down the steps of the dug-out. There was also some vague idea that he ought to have gone and seen whether he could help the sergeant or not, after he had been picked up and taken down the line. With the recognition that he was not in any way to blame for the incident and the death of the sergeant, he recovered from his repression, and lost certain of his neurotic symptoms.

Freud believes that certain symbols in dreams cannot be explained by the patient, and that these occur with considerable constancy in various people's dreams. He regards such symbols as fixed in their meaning, and believes that their interpretation is to be found by the study of myths and folklore. He argues from this that they are drawn from race memory rather than from individual memory, and that this explains why the individual cannot furnish an explanation. As has been said, great caution must be observed in regarding any given symbol as being of fixed significance. Be that as it may, there is no doubt that the study of any individual's dreams may throw considerable light on the constitution and working of his personality which might otherwise be misinterpreted. It might not be too much to say, that in evaluating any person, for any particular purpose, a systematic study of his dreams would be by no means without value.

Another important feature in relation to the working of the mind, on which Freud has laid stress, is what he calls the omnipotence of thought. By this he means that the individual attributes a value to purely cognitive processes quite out of proportion to reality. He recognizes this as an important constituent in the mentalities of the primitive, the child and the neurotic. Primitive man, so far as we can judge from observations on the low grade peoples who seem most closely to represent the behaviour of our ancestors, gradually evolved concepts of the supernatural, through the systems of taboo and magic. By the various processes of magic they believe that they can influence persons and things at a distance. These ideas of magic are closely allied to the early animism from which we have by no means yet freed ourselves, though we apply it much less widely, than did primitive man. The latter peopled the world with beneficent and maleficent spirits, and every person and object was possessed of a spirit, which could detach itself from the "body" and influence other "bodies" far removed in space. Freud points out that "Animism" is a system of thought, and it gives, not only the explanation of a single phenomenon, but makes it possible to comprehend the totality of the world from one point, as a continuity. He considers that animism grew out of the desire of man to master his surroundings. For this purpose he invented magic, and to explain magic he evolved animism. One process of magic is described by Frazer as imitative, that is to say, the savage performed some action similar to the end he desired, and believed that thereby this end was accomplished. The other process he described as contagious, and involved the treatment of some part or attribute (such as the name) of the object, which the savage desired to affect. This treatment involved, according to primitive belief, the experience by the object of just such dignities or indignities, as were practised on the part or attribute of the object. As Frazer says "Men mistook the order of their ideas for the order of their nature, and hence imagined that the control which they have, or seem to have, over their thoughts, permitted them to have a corresponding control over things." As Freud points out, Frazer's "order of their ideas" corresponds to the "order of their wishes," that these wishes if not gratified in reality, were gratified by hallucinations, which were of course believed as if they were real.

Similar reactions occur in the child. He finds himself at a disadvantage in gratifying his wishes in reality, and finds a ready gratification in hallucination. In young children, and also in older deficient children, an entirely undue valuation is put upon thought, and what the child wills to think, he believes is so. Adults are often apt to regard the results of this gratification by hallucination as deliberate lying, but when the imaginative child relates to an astonished parent how he met and vanquished a band of robbers, when out for his afternoon walk, he is not deliberately lying, he has only gratified his wish for self-assertion by an hallucination which he does not distinguish from reality. That he should be taught to distinguish between phantasy and reality, is of course necessary, but this may not be done best by abuse and punishment for telling lies. Similarly, the neurotic regresses very frequently to this level of being unable to distinguish between reality and phantasy, and having a firm belief in the identity of his wishes with accomplished fact. In the complete anamnesis of a neurotic patient, carried out by analytic methods, we are frequently astonished by tales of incidents which are said to have happened to the patient, but which further investigations prove to be entirely fictitious and merely "wish fulfilments." Again we frequently find him suffering from endless remorse, which is traced to a "death wish," expressed for some person, and which results firstly, in a fear that this wish may really have hurt the object, and secondly as a compensation, in an overweening anxiety for that person's health. Again, it is found that the difficulty experienced by the neurotic in adapting himself to life, is due to the difficulty in distinguishing between the values of reality and of phantasy to the detriment of the former. These beliefs in the omnipotence of thought, and the automatic fulfilment of wishes, are by no means confined to the neurotic, and are of great importance in understanding the behaviour of the average citizen, especially if he has never completely freed himself from the phase, which Freud describes, as the autoerotic, when he himself is the most important object of his desires, and therefore his own personal wishes demand gratification. In such a case, it is easy to hallucinate attributes which he does not possess.

A further psychological principle, on which Freud has laid considerable stress, especially in relation to the compulsion neuroses, he terms the ambivalence of emotion. By this he means, that it is very frequently observed that an individual displays two opposite feelings to an object, round which he has formed a complex or a sentiment. These antagonistic feelings may be experienced consecutively, or almost simultaneously, and may be exemplified by such everyday concurrences, as the attraction and repulsion felt by so many people at witnessing a particularly risky acrobatic feat. As Freud points out, however, this ambivalence becomes more important when one of the pair of opposites is repressed and unconscious, while the other is conscious ; and this is specially evident in the ambivalent feeling of love and hate so often displayed by both the neurotic, and the so-called normal individual, in respect to other people, especially relations. Similarly the Sadistic and Masochistic trends often go together, and are often directed towards the same individual. In fact, all the opposite varieties of feeling, pleasure, pain, attraction and repulsion, excitement and relaxation may be felt for the same object, consecutively or simultaneously. This was recognized by orthodox psychology to a certain extent, but it was not applied in the sense that Freud has applied it, and to him must be given the credit of laying stress on this extremely important factor in the mental make-up of the average man. It is clear, moreover, that any such conflict of emotions with regard to an object, will not make for the stability of the sentiment that emerges, and this ambivalence of emotion is one of the most potent factors which determine instability and conflict.

In a recent contribution, Freud has considerably modified his attitude in respect of what has been described above as the pleasure principle. This involves the theory that the set of all wishes is towards an active attainment of pleasure by relaxation of tension, and that this attainment of pleasure in his original sense always involved the co-operation, either as adjuvants or antagonists, of other wishes and "reality" or environment. Behind this, however, Freud thinks that any given wish has a tendency to return to its original condition, irrespective of the environment. This concept, he contends, involves a tendency of the individual as a whole to regress continually, until the original condition of non-existence or death is attained. For him then, life and progress are the products of reaction with reality, rather than fundamental "ends in view." These somewhat metaphysical concepts are admittedly vague, but they are suggestive as explaining to some extent the general phenomenon of regression, and some cases of suicide.

Recently, the Freudians have been engaged in the study of character, and have sought to demonstrate types based on the theories of regression and infantile fixations. They maintain that in the infant, the sex feeling is aroused by stimulus from areas outside the genital zone, specially from the mouth, anus and urethra, and that in some children, one or other of these extragenital erogenous zones are more than usually potent. When this is so, such children tend to grow up with specialized character traits, which owe much to fixation and regression, and to behaviour dependent on oral, anal, or urethral eroticism. These studies of character are not very clearly defined, except in the case of the so-called Anal-erotic, who corresponds in some degree, to the introvert sensational type, described in the next chapter. Such a man is avaricious and miserly, seeking to acquire and hoard wealth, neglectful of his own personal appearance and slovenly in his behaviour. Often he is childish and petulant, but loving childish things and toys, and sometimes he displays great love for children, but otherwise is unsociable and difficult. Arnold Bennett has displayed just this type in *Riceyman Steps*. Why such a character should be connected with anal eroticism, is by no means clear, and it is better to leave the explanation to the Freudians themselves, and reference should be made for this to their work. However, the fact remains, that they have successfully delineated a type of personality which may be met with in definite form from time to time.

As the Jungian character types seem more satisfactory, it is unnecessary to pursue this enquiry further at this point.

We have seen that many of the doctrines enunciated by Freud and his school are of great use in the study of Personality, but they ought to be used with care and discrimination. In criticizing the doctrines of Freud the chief point at issue is the loose use of terms. For example, the followers of Freud talk as if consciousness was a dynamic force which does things. Thus Dr Douglas Bryan,[7] in what purports to be a didactic article on psychoanalysis, says: "In general, it may be said that consciousness chooses what is pleasurable and avoids what is painful." There is absolutely no justification for investing consciousness with this power of choosing or of exerting any influence on mental processes. As Professor Woodbridge expresses it, consciousness is a state comparable to time and space, and just as we talk about things happening in time and in space we can talk about things happening in consciousness. This corresponds with the position taken up in this book, that consciousness involves a certain relatedness, and conscious phenomena are emergent resultants of this relatedness. Similarly "the unconscious" must be regarded as a state which involves life but does not enjoy that relatedness which we describe as consciousness, and we must not describe the unconscious as doing this or that. It is however, legitimate to consider certain patterns which may be unconscious or may be conscious. In considering such patterns it is necessary to deal with the primary concepts which form the basis of the Freudian argument, the sex complex or pattern, and the ego complex. Many Freudian writers imply that the only "impulse" which underlies behaviour is sex, and that this sex impulse is already active in infancy. They say that from birth till about five years of age almost any sensory stimulus activates this "impulse;" and that the resultant activity is "obviously" sexual. Thus von Hug-Helmuth[8] describes the muscular activity of a baby kicking his limbs about as resulting in the general excitement, the brightness of eyes, etc., which is in every way comparable to the behaviour of an adult in a sexual orgasm. Arguing in this way they talk of skin eroticism, muscle eroticism and mucous membrane eroticism, as the primary forms of sex activity. Then they recognize that certain areas of the body are established as special erogenous zones, such as the mouth, anus, genitalia, etc. These at first have equal selective activity for stimuli, and all lead to sexual activity, i.e., "sexual" feeling and "sexual" action. Later, under ordinary circumstances, the special zones, with the exception of the genitalia, lose their potency more or less and so the normal erotic sensation is confined to the proper physiological sexual system. Under special circumstances, however, the genitalia do not achieve complete predominance but this is shared or usurped by one or other of the erogenous zones, with the result that various perversions arise and, as has been mentioned above, special character traits are developed. However, it is not only on the receptive side that infantile sex is manifested, but also on the conative side, and the infant is said to have various wishes or sets towards muscular activity which are of a sexual nature. These are described under the headings of sadism, masochism, exhibitionism, prying, as well as the apparently more obviously sexual activities of embracing, cuddling, etc.

If we examine these on a physiological basis, two questions occur to us. Are these impulses sexual at all and can we usefully talk about impulses in this vague way without making any attempt to define what we mean by impulse, and how and from where the "driving force" of these impulses comes that we hear so much about. The primary forms of so-called eroticism are evidently undifferentiated sensory experience. That is to say, simple afferent patterns, which are not discriminated in the degree proper to fully developed cortical function, are activated by simple stimuli. For example, suppose an infant's skin is gently stroked, or the mucous membrane of his lips and gums are gently rubbed, a stimulus is applied which will activate certain afferent sensory neurone paths. If the stimulus is not too violent the activation will travel from the sensory neurones to certain vegetative neurones, with the result that glandular and smooth muscle activities will result, which are familiar to us as expressions of pleasure. At the same time certain striped muscle activities are manifested, which at this age are poorly integrated and for the most part ineffectual, but which have the general tendency of bringing the child into a position to receive more of the pleasant stimulus. Directly the stimulus passes a certain intensity it involves unpleasant feeling, and totally different behaviour results. Such behaviour resulting from purely sensory stimuli is characteristic of infancy, for with one exception, the patterns involved soon become more complicated and differently integrated. This complication of pattern and the differentiation of specific sensory experiences will result in a relative diminution of vegetative activity, and consequently in a diminished intensity of feeling, and an enhanced predominance of thought and integrated muscular activity. In consequence, this generalized indiscriminated excitement is not as a rule met with in the adult in response to the ordinary sensory stimulus. But there is an exception to this statement. The sex pattern is relatively late in its manifestation, and in the physical sex act there is retained, in adult life, a type of behaviour closely similar to that which is exhibited in response to the primary "sensational" experience, which is common in infantile life. Hug-Helmuth may be correct in stating that she has observed in the kicking infant who is enjoying kinesthetic sensation, behaviour similar to that of the adult enjoying sexual sensation, but it is suggested that she is wrong in deducing from this that the kinesthetic or tactile sensation of the infant is a sexual sensation; things which are examples of the same principle are not themselves identical. In his later works, Freud defines the sex impulses as those which tend to bring the individual into contact with an object of the environment, and doubtless the child is trying to do this, but it seems rather far fetched to call such an ill-defined series of impulses sexual, and identify them with adult sexuality. The special erogenous zones described by the Freudians are apparently those areas of the body in which the sensory end organs are most abundant and most specialized, and they are not inherently sexual in the adult sense. One of the arguments on which the Freudians base their claim to the truth of their concepts is that it affords an excellent explanation of the development of the perversions, and explains many symptoms of the neuroses, and that even in the normal adult, stimulation of the "erogenous zones" induces a more or less sexual experience. These contentions can, however, be adequately met by the concept of conditioning of patterns. It may well be that, as a result of hereditary or environmental influences, one or more of these patterns associated with sensory stimuli may become associated closely with the sex pattern and thus take on a definitely sexual association, although it was not originally sexual itself. This is normally the case with the stimulus to the mucous membrane of the mouth involved in kissing. This may go much further so that the whole sex pattern is modified and altered, so that an abnormal stimulus sets it off and a perversion results. Thus, suppose some sensory pattern Y, with stimulus X and activity Z, is brought into association with the sex pattern B, with normal stimulus A and activity C, the two may be so conditioned that instead of two processes taking place

only one process takes place thus,

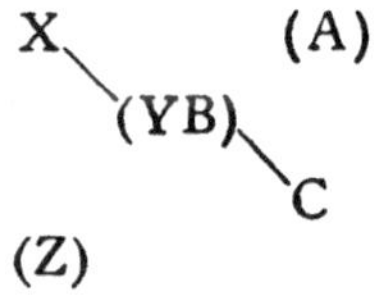

and A no longer activates any pattern, and the activity Z is no longer produced by any stimulus. This of course represents the extreme degree of a perversion, as for example, when ordinary sexual stimuli (A) have no effect whatever, while cruelty stimuli (X) actually produce orgasm (C) and do not in any degree produce the ordinary results (Z); but all intermediate processes occur, and are not uncommon. With regard to the conative tendencies mentioned above, there seems no particular reason to describe them as essentially sexual. In fact to do so would seem to be the result of arguing from the wrong end. No one will deny that sadism and masochism, exhibitionism, prying, and the like, as seen in adults are associated with sex, but the reason for this is that the very nature of the sex act demands that the sex pattern shall incorporate certain of these patterns as part of its complex whole. The sexual act being painful on the first occasion, it is necessary that a certain degree of active cruelty and submission to cruelty should be exhibited, and in certain cases the normal sex pattern may be profoundly modified and even totally submerged by the sadistic or masochistic pattern, if these are strongly developed. This will lead to perversions, but it is nothing but another example of conditioning. For instance, the small boy who pulls the wings off flies is not doing anything sexual, but later on his sex pattern may be conditioned by this pattern, which subserves cruel behaviour, so that he becomes a sexual sadist. At first sight exhibitionism and prying, seem to be more definitely sexual even in infancy, but it must be remembered that these types of behaviour are closely associated with curiosity, and that in consequence they will be concerned not with the obvious, but with those things which custom keeps hid. Young children will often exhibit or "pry into" their sexual organs, but equally often they will concern themselves with micturition or defecation, which cannot reasonably be regarded as sexual acts, but they have this in common that they are all usually hidden from observation. To sum up this argument, it would appear that the Freudians, who derive all sorts of manifestations from sexuality, are making the same mistake as those earlier critics of Darwinism who pointed to the monkey in the zoo as their friends' great-grandfather, oblivious of the fact that Darwin postulated a common ancestry to monkey and man ; so it would appear that sexual experience is only one form of primary sensory experience, and the sexual "wish" is only one form of the primary infantile wishes, and that the perversions are not primary, but develop secondarily through conditioning. It is necessary also, to realize the development of the sexual impulse. Based on the impulse to physical satisfaction, the pattern soon gets involved with other impulses whose end in view is not physical satisfaction at all. Freud's explanation that love is made up of impulses which are not inhibited, comprising sensual love, and similar impulses which are inhibited, comprising spiritual love or tenderness, hardly seems to meet the case. Freud would derive all the components of the love sentiment from the physical impulse, which is the original "instinct" of sex in the predisposition, using the word instinct in McDougall's sense. The latter is right in protesting against the practice of the Freudians in mixing up parental instinct and sex instinct, as if they were one and the same thing, at the level of the predisposition ; but there can be no doubt that with the advance of life, they do become integrated together, and condition each other, so that it becomes difficult to separate them. It is always difficult to analyse such a complex sentiment as love, but in his treatment of this sentiment McDougall lays stress on the grouping of emotional reactions in relation to the object, and exemplifies this by describing the anger when the object is attacked, fear when she is in danger, and so forth. Yet there is more in love than this, and it is suggested that there is an aspect of love with which McDougall does not deal and which the Freudians make use of, but without any exact definition or analysis. Roughly we may define love as an attraction between two people; what then are the elements of attraction between these two? This attraction can best be understood if three factors are distinguished. Firstly, physical appetite; secondly, possession, an impulse to take; and thirdly the parental feeling, the desire to protect, the impulse to give. These are combined in the way which we suggest all biological units are combined, that is, so as to give rise to a new emergent having an identity of its own, and quite distinguishable from its components. The first needs no description here. The second is the basis of jealousy if carried too far, and is characterized by the wish that the object shall belong exclusively to the subject, that he or she shall minister to the needs and desires of the subject, and sacrifice himself and herself for the sake of the subject. This is the attitude which too often becomes dominant after marriage. Like other affective reactions, up to a certain intensity, it is desirable and attractive; but if excessive, it is undesirable and repulsive. The third factor, that of the parental impulse, involves a sacrifice of self, a giving out in the interests of the object. It is entirely antithetical to the last and frequently comes into conflict with it. It is perhaps most marked in the woman, but it is noticeable that, at any rate so far as courtship is concerned, the woman in whom this self-denying factor is dominant is by no means the most attractive to the opposite sex.

If we now consider the various attractions which exist between human beings we can recognize how these three factors are represented, and we may illustrate what is meant to greater advantage. Between lovers of the opposite sex, all three should be so integrated that they assume a true fusion without conflict. Ideally, the first will enter into the attraction without obtruding itself, the second will be present in each, to such an extent as to satisfy the third impulse in the other, and the third will similarly be reciprocal to the demands of the second in the partner. If the first is too strong in one, or too weak in the other, to be reciprocal to the requirements of each other, there will be friction; and it is obvious that the second and third, being the antithesis of each other, must be reciprocal. Even the third will do harm if in excess, though at first sight it seems so desirable; for no man, or woman either, likes to be fussed over more than a certain amount. These second and third factors are not of course inversely proportionate, for a man may have an almost unlimited capacity for receiving from his mate and yet be capable of giving much himself. Results of incompatibility of the three factors are so obvious that discussion is unnecessary, but incompleteness or completeness of the love sentiment is clearly an important factor in the development of personality.

In the attraction between parent and child, the third factor should be the dominant one, and while the child is young it usually is so, corresponding to the unlimited capacity for taking, on the part of the child. But very soon the child himself begins to develop this third impulse and may play upon the second in the parent, so that by the time the child is grown up the relative positions may be reversed. If the parental impulse is ideal, the giving must be for the ultimate good of the object, and if carried on too long may subtly change to the second impulse of taking. The cat, who after a time turns her kittens out and refuses them further protection and care, is not a hard-hearted mother, but is acting wisely for the future of her offspring; we may thus describe for a moment what is an irrational instinctive action, as if it were conscious in the human sense. But the human mother, who ties her children to her apron-strings in the belief that she is a perfect mother, and while protecting them from harm, is really indulging her possessive impulse, is taking and not giving. In spite of what many Freudians say it is improbable that the first factor is of any significance in the average relationship of parent and child, though to contend that it never occurred, would be untrue. But the tragedies that occur as a result of disproportion between the second and third factors are legion.

In the relationship of friends, the first factor is unimportant or non-existent, though in many so-called friendships this is not so entirely absent as the subjects would like to believe. The third factor should be dominant, and the second present in slight degree, but too often the latter becomes obtrusive and results in jealousies and discord. We may conclude, then, that the Freudian use of the term sex is too indiscriminated, and leads to too great a simplification of the springs of behaviour, even between normal lovers.

We have complained above, that Freud paid too little attention to the self-preservation impulses, and, indeed, in his earlier works Freud was somewhat vague about the ego complex, and grouped the instincts which specially subserved self-preservation under this head, without analysing them particularly. He regarded these tendencies as chiefly concerned in conflicting with sex, and along with the reality principle, repressing and censoring the sexual tendencies, so as to constitute defences and reactions against the activities of the latter. Later, however, he and his followers describe a state of development of the sex "libido" which is directed to the ego itself, which they term Narcissism. This stage may be recognized in early infancy in the normal individual, and may persist as a fixation in the abnormal. In this case there is no striving outwards towards an object, since the subject itself has become the object. More recently still, Freud has taken up the study of the ego complex itself, and he insists that the effort of seeking the object is the reaction with the environment which involves life, and therefore the group of instincts which set the individual towards this may be termed life instincts. These he identifies with his sex complex. On the other hand, there are a group of instincts which set the individual away from the object in the environment, whose purpose is to shelter him from contact with the environment, to the maintenance and encouragement of which the whole effort of the individual is directed in the narcissistic stage. This withdrawal from the object, in Freud's view, involves a retiral from life and a constant tendency to revert to the simplest and least exacting contact with the environment, i.e., to a Nirvana state, with its logical outcome in non-existence, or death. This group of instincts he therefore terms the death instincts, and identifies them with the ego complex. This will naturally be in conflict with the sex or life instincts, and may therefore lead to fixations and repressions. In Freud's view, the narcissistic phase is not a true expression of these instincts, and does not lead to death, because there is even in this, a striving outwards for an object, i.e. towards life, but the object is identified with the ego. That the ego is objective and not subjective, is shown by the fact, that there may be a well-marked division between the ego and the ego ideal, between what the individual is and what he would like to be, and to this he is striving. When this division is sharp and deep, the individual feels depressed and melancholic, whereas when the difference is slight, there is self-satisfaction, culminating in the extreme "pleasure" characteristic of mania when the ego and ego ideal fuse.

The true ego complex, according to Freud's presentation, may be defined as that group of impulses which tend to foster the interests and satisfactions of the self, as opposed to those of any object outside the self. It will tend to be in opposition to any effort to find contact for any purpose or in any way, with an object in the environment. As the outcome of this tendency must be towards Nirvana or non-existence, these tendencies never can find complete satisfaction during life, and so will manifest themselves rather as negative restricting influences than positive influences achieving any definite activity of themselves. Such in the main is Freud's view, but it is questionable whether the ego may not be more positive in its activities than this attitude represents. The ego cannot remain detached and as development proceeds, more and more of the environment is merged in the ego and a better presentation of the ego development would seem to be the self-regarding sentiment, as described by McDougall, and referred to in Chapter VII.

Those activities of an individual which involve contact with an object outside of himself for any purpose whatever, are katabolic; while those which protect him from this contact, are anabolic. If then, the sex complex in Freud's sense comprises the tendencies which make for contact with the environment, they may be based on the various katabolic agencies of the body, sympathetic nervous system, thyroid, pituitary, adrenal group of endocrine organs, and so forth. On the other hand, if the ego complex comprises the tendencies which make for avoidance of contact with the object, they may be based on the anabolic agencies, the autonomic nervous system, the pancreatic endocrine group, and so on. But anabolism is not merely a negative process of avoidance of katabolism, but a positive process in itself. Hence it would seem probable that there is a definite ego "libido" in addition to the sex "libido" or, as we should prefer to express it, the ego complex may be just as much a definite engraphic pattern, capable of being activated, as is the sex complex. Therefore, the former may be modified by the reality principle, and such modification may result in conflict with the environment, just as much as may the latter. If we are to accept this rough analogy of anabolic and katabolic tendencies, it is clear that they are antithetic to each other and are continually in a state of conflict. Such conflict may be resolved by compromise or one or other may be temporarily suppressed, one or other may be conscious or unconscious, and the engrams which subserve these complexes will vary from time to time in their constitution, and their relatedness will differ, so that they may or may not achieve consciousness. It follows then that the relatedness which involves consciousness is a property of the constellation or complex, rather than that a constellation is the property of consciousness, as Freudians sometimes appear to infer. Some critics seem tempted to ask whether this conception does not involve the premise that once any mental process has been integrated on the level of consciousness, it must always remain there; whereas the Freudian psychologists, if they are right, have shown that many things, which have been conscious at one time cease to be so. But this contention would not be held by the philosophers of emergent evolution at all; on the other hand, they would be ready to admit that the integration at the conscious level is a much less stable affair than, for example, integration at the level of life. When we rise to the level of consciousness we have to do with the series of integrations which are essentially unstable, and which do not necessarily persist for any length of time. Not only may constellations become unconscious, but, at the level of consciousness, their complexity and relatedness may vary considerably. As Professor Janet[4] has so well shown, the individual is constantly running up and down the scale of integrations on these higher levels. He points out that individuals vary to an enormous extent in the energy which they have at their command for carrying out their actions; and that the same individual varies in the amount of energy he has at his disposal from day to day, and hour to hour. But if we are considering behaviour, we are at once struck by two different aspects of any action carried out—the amount of energy which is put into it, and its efficiency in relation to the environment. As Hughlings Jackson pointed out, an epileptic fit is no more than a manifestation of low grade motor activity released from higher control, and if we compare the behaviour of a man in an epileptic fit with that of a man going for a walk, we may possibly give the prize for energy to the man in the fit, though we shall certainly give the prize for efficiency to the man going for a walk. Janet expresses this phenomenon as follows:—At lower levels, energy is expended at once, whereas, at higher levels, it may be capitalized and put into reserve. This capitalization allows the individual, not only to modify his immediate environment in time and space, but to extend that influence through time and space. Simple minds can carry on their work from day to day and are, at the most, capable of preparing their nourishment for to-morrow, but the superior man can integrate his actions so as to modify human life for many years. Founding his argument on this basis, he attempts to describe a hierarchy of levels of behaviour, according to the extensiveness of their power of action in time and space. As we ascend this hierarchy of levels, behaviour becomes much more complex in reality, though at first sight it may seem simple enough. Directly behaviour reaches the actively conscious level the influence of self-consciousness comes in. Directly it reaches the level of social behaviour, the influence of consciousness of other people comes in, and the more remote these people are, and the more behaviour is directed, with regard, not only to the opinion of contemporaries but to that of future generations, the more complex the reactions become. The more recent tendencies and the more complicated and higher levels of behaviour, are the least stable in any individual; and it is in this respect that the study of the neurasthenic becomes so useful for normal psychology, because in him we can see the effect of the absence of the higher levels of integration; just as at lower levels, we can study the effect of absence of motor and sensory cortical control, by examining patients with lesions of the sensory and motor cortex. From this we can see, therefore, that there is no objection to the concept of the interplay of life and death impulses, of sex and ego, as described by Freud, one assuming the ascendancy at one time, and the other at another, under the influence of successive inhibitions and facilitations. But we must realize that the consciousness or unconsciousness of these impulses is a function of themselves, and that they are not extruded from consciousness or erupted from the unconscious state, by some mysterious force which breaks through the "censor." This being so, another criticism of Freudian terminology follows. Just as they talk of consciousness doing things, so they talk of the censorship doing things. So long as the censor is simply regarded as a concept, and used for the purpose of describing a series of more or less complicated physio-psychological processes of inhibition, there may be no harm in this, if we are anxious to dramatize the presentation of our concepts. But again to quote Dr Douglas Bryan who says: "This barrier is a repressing force, which is constantly exerting itself, to prevent the contents of the true unconscious from reaching consciousness, their contents striving as they do, in order to obtain an outlet through consciousness, to discharge the energy with which they are invested." When we come across a sentence like this, we begin to ask ourselves what this censor is, and we may be tempted to enquire where we are going to find it in our anatomical and physiological studies. It may be all right for the accomplished Freudian, who knows exactly how the concept of the censorship was arrived at, but the article from which this sentence is quoted is supposed to be for the young beginner, and such a neophyte would surely think from this that the censor was some definite entity, related somehow or other to some brain structure. As we have seen, the censor is only a highly speculative term used to describe the effects of the inhibition of activation, comparable to such physiological manifestations as are exemplified by the inhibition of the antagonist muscles by the agonists, in the movement of a limb, the suppression of the mass spinal reflex by higher level activity, and the fusion of motor activity controlled by the prespinal arc with that controlled by the pyramidal system. To sum up, there does not seem any inherent difference between such mutual incompatibility and mutual repressions of agonists and antagonists, or the mutually inhibitive action of the sphincter and compressor muscles of a hollow viscus and the mutually repressive action of sex and ego complexes. Again, the repression of the mass reflex, which is only revealed when all higher controlling influences are removed, is comparable to certain archaic racial dispositions only showing themselves in extreme cases of regression, which represent a marked state of devolution of the higher forms of relatedness. The suppression of certain movements useful at one stage of life, such as the active sucking of the lips on contact, is of the same nature as the repression of early experiences which, as life advances, become painful or regressive in their influence. Again, it is not uncommon for us to repress wittingly childish habits of movement in walking or other motions, and this is comparable to the repression of painful incidents, distinguished by Rivers. Finally, the fusion of prespinal and pyramidal motor activity, so that the perfect motility of the healthy animal may emerge, would seem to be comparable to the fusion of various dispositions to constitute a sentiment, such as love, as has been described above. Such are a few of the criticisms and amendments which might be advanced in connexion with Freud's work, but there can be no question that he has made a contribution to the study of personality of the utmost value. Though no doubt much has still to be worked out, and many of his original contentions may require modification, his insistence on the importance of conflict and repression at psychological levels, and his study of their results, will one day be found to be in strict correlation with the work done on conflicts and repressions at physiological levels, and even in his apparently more contentious concepts, loose terminology is apparently the chief difficulty we have to contend with, and it may be that if an adequate translation into scientific terms can be obtained, these will not seem so far-fetched as they frequently do at present.

CHAPTER X

THE CONTRIBUTION OF JUNG TO THE STUDY OF PERSONALITY

FROM the purely psychological standpoint we find that the line of thought adopted in this book is in sympathy with the attitude of Jung,[1] when he broke away from the strict Freudian school. In the first place, he recognized that the general set of man's life was directed to an achievement of something higher, to something creative, to Deity in Alexander's sense. Jung saw that the aim was not merely the achievement of sexual desire, or even of love, or of individual expression, as Freud and Adler, respectively, would have us believe. However, as was said in Chapter VIII, all these theories are complementary rather than mutually destructive. As to the means whereby this end is achieved, however, we would find ourselves at variance with Jung as he, like Freud, postulates a libido comparable to the *élan vital* of Bergson, coming from somewhere outside, and being of a different order to the ordinary processes of physiology.

Secondly, we find ourselves in sympathy with Jung's treatment of the word sex. While we have found it necessary to criticize the application of the term sex to much in infantile behaviour, Jung criticizes the too free use of the term in later developments. He maintains that, though many processes in the behaviour of mankind may have developed from sexual conations, nevertheless, in their fully established state, they ought not to be described as sexual, since they are permanently changed. In other words, an emergence from sexual and other conations in combination is no longer sexual, but something new and distinctive in virtue of its emergence.

To turn to the actual contribution of Jung to the study of personality, it is not within the scope of this work to consider the whole of his teaching as it relates to the practice of psychotherapy, but there are certain aspects of his philosophy which are of the greatest importance to our particular study.

The two outstanding features of Jung's contribution are his concept of a collective unconscious, and his scheme of differentiation into types. Jung approached the study of human personality from the same avenue as did Freud, namely through the symptoms of the abnormal mind, and only later was he led to the study of the behaviour of the normal individual. Neither of these observers interested himself primarily, as did the American school, with the physiological applications of this approach, but confined themselves entirely to the psychological aspect of the problem. Nevertheless, as Jung himself has pointed out, the objects of their investigation and the interpretation of their findings were divergent from the outset, and must have been so, because they belong to different types, who could not see the problem from the same standpoint It is necessary to examine these differences further, before we proceed. Freud, the extrovert, was interested in the object, in what he could successively find, and describe as objective facts, by deeper and deeper analysis. Thus, he observed psychic traumata on the one hand, and the behaviour of his patient on the other, and inferred that the former had a causal relation to the latter. Jung, the introvert, was interested in how all these discoveries applied to the subject from the standpoint, not of the observer, but of the subject himself. This led him to suspect some of the inferences of Freud, and to formulate different causal relationships to explain behaviour. Any situation must be regarded as a complex from which we have no right to detach, either the contribution of the object, or that of the subject, and we must investigate it from both points of view before we can grasp the situation as a whole. Take a simple example. I am hit by a falling rock which breaks my arm. The extravert, in examining this situation, would be concerned with an empirical investigation of the facts. He would first treat the rock as an object, he would observe that it became detached from the mountain, that it fell through a certain space, that it struck my arm and bounded off to drop at my feet. Then he would observe me, and describe how my arm was struck, how I uttered a cry, and how my arm fell useless. From this, he would infer inductively, that I felt pain, and that my arm was broken, because experience of similar objective observances told him that this explanation was most likely. The attitude which the introvert would take is more difficult to describe, because our language does not lend itself so easily to this type of thought. This introvert attitude is not readily appreciated or accepted by the Anglo-Saxon mind, or indeed, by the Western mind at all, for introversion is much more general in the Oriental. Such an observer would tend to identify himself with the situation as subject. He would consider how I felt, and to do this, must to a certain extent put himself in my place. He would be interested in how I, as a subject, reacted to the event; what contribution I, as subject, made to the complex situation. He would not necessarily conclude that I suffered pain, and that my arm was broken because, as the extravert would say, "It was perfectly obvious that it was." He might consider the possibility that I had an anæsthetic arm, and so might not have had any pain, and that the cry was evoked by surprise at the noise of the stone falling. He might weigh the possibility that my arm fell to my side, not because it was broken, but only because it was bruised; he would be less interested in the facts than in possible explanations. Though he might, and probably would come to the same general conclusion as the extravert, he would only arrive at it after considering and rejecting other possibilities. Similarly, if he considered the stone as subject, he would identify himself, so far as possible, with it, and be interested less in the fact that it fell than in the laws which determined its fall. Carried to extremes, this attitude is prone to anthropomorphize objects, in the manner of the primitive man; and such would attribute to the stone, for instance, a feeling and cognition of falling, almost a consciousness of situation in time and space which, to the extravert mind, is a *reductio ad absurdum*. I have purposely given a somewhat crude and exaggerated example, but I wish to make clear that in a given complex situation, the extravert is concerned with the contribution to the situation of the objects, as objects-of-observation, while the introvert is interested in the subject and his subjective experiences, quite apart from what happens to him. So in the study of behaviour, Freud was concerned with what happened to the individual who was being studied, and what his reaction was, in strict relationship to this happening. He therefore took notice of the psychic traumata experienced by the individual, he saw the reactions induced by these, and formulated his contribution, which is described elsewhere, laying stress on behaviour as a function of the stimulus, though admitting the influence of disposition.

Jung, on the other hand, saw what the individual contributed of himself and from himself, laying stress on behaviour as a function of the disposition, though not denying the influence of stimuli. From this standpoint he came to the conclusion that there was, in each individual mind, a store of potential reactions to stimuli, which have no fundamental relation to his own experience or to environment, though they may be modified by these. He suggests that they are in fact the expressions of primitive race experience, which give the individual an inner set towards meeting a situation in the way the race has been accustomed to meet it. Such a set is analogous to the behaviour of the heart, which, in virtue of its structural and functional organization, has a set towards responding to the needs of the body to be nourished by circulating blood. Further, he suggests, quite apart from any experience or influence from the environment, that in accordance with the variations in these dispositions and their interrelations, there is a tendency for individuals to respond to the situations met with in life, in certain different ways. These he has distinguished in his eight types.

To get a complete understanding of his concepts it is necessary to have recourse to his own works, and those of his apologists, and it must suffice here to indicate briefly how they contribute to the study of personality.

First of all, we may study his conception of the collective unconscious. Jung defines the unconscious as an exclusively psychological concept. For him, the term covers all those psychic contents, or processes, which are not conscious, i.e., not related to the ego in a perceptible way. He justifies the concept of the existence of such contents on the evidence of psychopathological and other experience. Take, for instance, a case of hysterical amnesia; at any given moment, the ego knows nothing of the existence of certain complicated psychological complexes, and yet, in the next moment, a simple hypnotic procedure is enough to bring the lost contents to complete reproduction in consciousness. He holds that it is quite impossible to specify what contents the unconscious embraces; only experience can decide such questions. We may form general impressions, but cannot expect them to hold good in individual instances. Firstly the disappearance of a great variety of complexes which were once conscious in the process of forgetting, involves their presence as unconscious content, as is shown by their reappearance, sooner or later, by virtue of some new relatedness. Secondly, he considers that certain sense perceptions may, by reason of their slight intensity or because of the deviation of attention, scarcely reach that special relatedness which involves full consciousness, yet become unconscious psychic contents. Again, the existence of such contents may be demonstrated, inasmuch as they may be revealed under hypnosis. Finally, experience also teaches us that there exist unconscious psychic patterns—for instance, mythological images—which have never been in, or near consciousness during the individual's lifetime, and hence must have been engraphically determined, entirely at the level of unconscious activity. Thus, Jung would divide the content into two divisions of unconscious levels. Firstly, a personal unconscious, including that which has been forgotten and repressed, and that which represents subliminal impressions: in other words, all those patterns resulting from the interaction of the disposition with the environment which have failed to reach, or ceased to enjoy, that relatedness, which involves consciousness. Secondly, he describes the collective unconscious whose contents do not originate in personal acquisitions, but in the inherited potentiality of psychic function which is subserved by the inherited brain structure. This collective unconscious material consists of the mythological primordial images—those motives and images, which apparently can spring anew in every age and clime, without historic tradition or personal migration. There are many examples, especially in the history of symbols, which seem to bear this out; for example, the universality of the serpent and fish symbols for fertility, and the attitude of primitives to the four elementals, earth, air, fire and water. Again, in art, there are many similarities in the work of artists of different periods, which are difficult to explain on the basis of culture contact, though, in most cases this cannot be absolutely excluded. Examples might be quoted, such as that of the three-dimensional feeling of the negroid art, which has recently been to the fore in artistic circles, compared to the same feeling in Greek art. Again, compare certain recently discovered examples of Minoan art from Crete, with Masaccio's "Expulsion from the garden of Eden" in the Carmine chapel in Florence, and that, in turn, with the modern work of Degas. Or in poetry, the analytical but hyperbolic verse of Donne in England, with that of his contemporary Gongora, in Spain. All these may serve to show that in the absence of obvious common environmental influences, similar behaviour patterns emerge, as if from a common source. Just as conscious content is integrated and combined to produce behaviour in the form of conscious actions and thought, so unconscious content is integrated and combined on a different level of relatedness, to produce overt behaviour in the form of unconscious actions and thought processes, such as appear in dreams or phantasies. This does not imply that any content which at times enjoys the special relatedness which involves consciousness takes no part in such actions and dreams; but rather, that their set and pattern depend chiefly on that content which does not enjoy such relatedness, and so is unconscious. This, of course, refers to activities and thoughts, which Jung would place in that division of unconscious mental activity which he calls the collective unconscious, for most of the content of the individual unconscious mind has, at one time or another, enjoyed the relatedness which involves consciousness.

Jung further regards the unconscious content as compensatory; that is to say, when there is a gap in the stream of proper conscious content which would enable the subject to deal adequately with a situation, this gap is filled by unconscious content. But, inasmuch as this latter content has failed to achieve that higher relatedness which we call consciousness, its adaptation to environment is primitive and incomplete, and therefore more or less unsatisfactory. It follows from this that the more one-sided is the conscious content, the more obviously compensatory will be the unconscious content, a factor which will be noticed further when dealing with the dissociated personality, and conscious and unconscious behaviour will be complementary to each other. Thus, in relation to the types of introvert and extravert already discussed; if an individual is a marked extravert in his conscious behaviour, his unconscious behaviour will tend to be of the introverted type, and vice versa. Hence, in dealing with neurotics, whose behaviour is largely of the poorly integrated and discriminated unconscious type, their real category is frequently mistaken, since their most obvious behaviour is really compensatory and not genuine.

So far as this view of the unconscious content is concerned, there is no difficulty in accepting most of it from the physiological point of view, so long as we remember that the content of the collective unconscious can only be described as existing in certain relationships. There has been far too much talk on the part of some writers, about the collective unconscious doing this and that; a confusion of thought which cannot be too much deprecated. As has been said above, the most original part is the concept that the collective unconscious is the basis of a purely subjective contribution to a situation which has nothing to do with objective experience. The crucial points in this theory of the existence of race memories in the individual psychic content are as follows: firstly, we must admit the possibility of transmission of particular patterns of behaviour which we recognize as the common actions of our ancestors, at some time or other, speaking of such as correlates of special patterns of neural structure; secondly, if such patterns are transmitted, we must explain how they may be available for use under a certain concatenation of circumstances.

We have accepted Semon's[2] theory of the Mneme, as a useful concept which seems to explain the facts and is, moreover, reasonably likely to approximate to the truth. This theory emphatically allows for the transmission of just such characters as Jung suggests. An engram is an arrangement of neurones, conditioned in such a way that their subsequent activation produces a pattern of behaviour which resembles, but is not identical with the previous resultant behaviour. Such engrams are evolved out of inherited dispositions, by the modification necessitated by the environment. It would seem that in this process of the evolution of engrams, two factors must be taken into account. The neural patterns or engrams are not only an imprint on a malleable material induced by the environment, as a crest is imprinted on soft wax by a signet-ring, but there is in that relatedness, which involves life, a tendency to achieve adaptation; and so, in respect of this, an engram will take on a certain form which subserves greater adaptability. In other words, it is not only a function of the environment, but also of that relatedness which involves life. This concept does not involve any special vital energy, but simply that the relatedness follows certain laws, and these laws imply behaviour which, if followed, will lead *to* adaptation rather than away from it. Recent experiments have shown that such engrams which are determined in the nervous system, and which become progressively adaptive in the individual animal, also by some modification of the germ cell are represented in the next generation, not in their original form, but in their later form of greater adaptability. Thus, it has been found that not only will an individual animal, learning by experience, require fewer and fewer trials and errors in finding its way out of a maze, but its offspring will learn more quickly than did the parent, and the diminution of trials and errors, necessary in the learning progress, will be transmitted through several generations. If this be so, then it may be admitted that engrams representing primitive patterns of thought and feeling, acquired during the life-time of various individuals, may be transmitted in their modified form to future generations.

On the analogy of motor activity, it is to be expected that such primitive patterns, which are transmitted, will be unconscious and not conscious. Thus Rivers[3] has pointed out how many functions, which are no longer necessary to the individual, may be either totally suppressed, or suppressed and fused. For example, it is certain that the type of locomotion which is represented in the central nervous system by the prespinal arc, was the actively functioning pattern of behaviour in a remote ancestor. In human beings it is suppressed below the level of consciousness, and below the level at which it can function independently; yet it is still an essential part of our motor organization; for if interfered with by disease or injury, or if allowed undue prominence by the cessation of the normal control exercised by the cortical motor system, locomotion is at once interfered with by the alteration of muscular tonus. So with these patterns of thought and feeling, described by Jung as the collective unconscious. They have been suppressed below the level of conscious relatedness, and only achieve activation when, in sleep or neurosis, the controlling and inhibitory influence of conscious mentality is in abeyance. This liberation from conscious control which allows these unconscious engrams to be activated, explains how they find expression at certain times, and therefore elucidates the second problem which we submitted for solution. To support this, it is noticeable that when these engrams are activated and achieve anything like dominance, the influence on the individual is usually a disturbing one. For all we know, however, their presence, though unconscious, may have a considerable influence on normal behaviour; in other words, they may be fused and not suppressed. This question cannot be fully determined till psychologists know a great deal more about subconscious mental processes. There seems no reason, then, to reject the contention of Jung, that our personality includes these primitive patterns of mental activity which can, under certain circumstances, be reactivated according to the Mnemic laws. Usually, however, like other superseded activities, they are suppressed below the level of consciousness. So they are not influenced by those constant modifications and changes which are impressed on our more conscious patterns by the reciprocal relationship of individual and environment. For this reason, their occasional manifestations will bear a close resemblance, even in individuals of very different types, and will likewise reproduce with considerable fidelity the habitual patterns of thought and feeling of primitive man. In other words, behaviour, depending on collective unconscious processes, is archaic and badly adapted.

When we come to consider Jung's other contribution to the study of the personality, viz., his differentiation of types, we must distinguish between his earlier and later work. Originally, he chose two types, the introvert and the extravert, which corresponded as he then described them, to the introverted thinking type and the extraverted feeling type of his new classification. The more elaborate classification of his later work is a distinct advance and removes several difficulties. In the first place, it relieves us from the necessity of postulating two definite types of introvert and extravert. He now defines introversion and extraversion as attitudes. The four types he relates to the four mental functions of thinking, feeling, intuition and sensation. Whichever of these functions is predominant in an individual determines his type, and this type will be introverted or extraverted according to his prevalent attitude towards his environment, which may vary from time to time; so that, although we may say that a person is an introvert, he may be extraverted towards certain objects, and at certain times. Thus a man may be introverted towards his religion, but extraverted towards his garden, while another may be extraverted in health, but become introverted during illness. Indeed, there are some extraverts who maintain that introversion is always pathological, and there is a good deal to be said in favour of such a view. None the less, there is no doubt that we can recognize in most people a dominant attitude and a recessive attitude, that is to say that most of the time the dominant attitude, either extravert or introvert prevails, and only under certain circumstances does the recessive attitude manifest itself. An attempt has already been made to indicate the contrast between extravert and introvert, and for fuller details reference should be made to Jung's own works. Similarly in respect of the types, it is impossible to do more than indicate their nature here. One fact, however, may be referred to. This is that the intuitive and sensation types, which Jung calls the irrational types but which would be better called the empirical types as Van der Hoop has suggested, would seem to represent a lower stage in the development of the personality than the thinking and feeling types. Following the strictly correlationist standpoint adopted in this study, we recognize that the functions of the cortex are the highest development so far attained by the brain of man. We have seen that the chief of these are integration, discrimination and control. The principal difference between the rational and empirical types is that the latter are content to accept the facts of life, or the impulses they feel within themselves, as they come. They have no desire to discriminate these, or integrate them into systems, or control them so that they come within the scope of rational laws, as do the former; and it is just these functions which are characteristic of full cortical development, and therefore are higher in the scale. For this reason I would not regard the functions of thinking and feeling, in the empirical types, as recessive, in the sense that sensation and intuition are recessive in the rational types. In the rational type, sensation and intuition have been superseded for general purposes but by no means suppressed, so that in certain situations intuition or sensation is the function that is called upon. On the other hand, in the empirical types, the functions of thinking and feeling have not yet come to full fruition, and so are only made use of tentatively and occasionally.

By the function of sensation, we mean that the normal sensations acquire a sufficient degree of relatedness to achieve consciousness, and form perceptions, but are not further integrated into abstract concepts or complicated emotional relationships. Under the term sensation we must include all sensations, whether the result of stimuli coming from the environment or from within the body. I retain the term sensation type because it has been used by Jung, and a multiplication of terms, referring to the same thing, is undesirable; but it seems to be a little unfortunate to use a term which has a perfectly definite meaning on one level, to express something indubitably dependent on what is expressed by the original term, but which has acquired a new relatedness, and has emerged at a higher level. For what the sensation type experiences are not pure sensations, but an organization of such, so that they emerge as perceptions. These perceptions might be described in our daily press, by the favourite adjective "sensational", for people of this type are apt to live at a high tension, passing from one "sensation" in the journalistic sense, to another. The contribution of their inherent impulses, irrespective of response to psychic traumata, is recessive, and only makes itself felt under exceptional circumstances. That is to say, they require something to which they can respond, before action is initiated. When their inherent impulses do initiate action, by breaking away from the usual channels of responses, such action is undiscriminated and uncontrolled, as it has not achieved that degree of relatedness which corresponds to full cortical or conscious control. That these people do behave, in response to accidents of the environment, in the way that Freud would have us believe, is practically universal; and their sex impulse, for instance, is either poorly controlled, or repressed by some stronger stimulus from the environment.

If the sensation type is extraverted, a man is specially sensitive to, and interested in stimuli from without. Such individuals often achieve considerable powers of discrimination in respect of these, and many artists are of this type, excelling in virtue of this sensory discrimination. As a rule, this type are of the class met with in scores at

English country houses, interested chiefly in sensuous pleasures in the broadest sense, which include the pleasures of muscular exercise and simple visual, auditory and gustatory stimuli, but they are restrained by tradition, which divides conduct into things which are "done", and the things which are "not done". This results in a very definite ethical code, arranged according to the dictates of this tradition, which does not always correspond to the Decalogue. Moreover, conduct is frequently dominated by that eleventh commandment, "Thou shalt not be found out." The thinking of these people is superficial, and the only realities for them are facts, and what they call "common sense". Abstractions and metaphysics are quite meaningless and simply a waste of time. Their feeling also tends to be superficial, they have hosts of acquaintances but do not readily make close friends. They say they are deeply moved by events, but alter their lives very little as the result of these "moving experiences", for their own emotions are not deeply fixed and are poorly organized, nor are they capable of real and lasting sympathy. Their chief recessive characteristic is the behaviour dictated by their own "wishes", which is characteristic of the intuitive type. Of this they are desperately afraid, because it usually cuts across the tradition by which they are guided, and leads to a state of confusion from which they see no outlet, owing to the poverty of their capacity for thought. Being a recessive character, the type of reaction is poorly discriminated and controlled, and tends too much to an "all or none" reaction. Hence they are liable at times to violent swings from one extreme to the other, between strictly conventional behaviour and that dictated by their primitive unconscious impulses,—behaviour which used to be described as "Mafeking".

If the sensation type is introverted, a man will be interested chiefly in the impressions he receives from within himself, and will react, even to outside stimuli, from this point of view, so that the resultant perception is dominated chiefly by the influence of the individual's store of images rather than by pure sense impressions. Much modern art is the product of this type. The only law that governs it is the expression of how the artist sees a thing. The resultant picture may be, and generally is very different from the photographic impression which the extravert of the same type would experience. Indeed, it may be that any other person would perceive the original as something entirely different, but this does not in any way disturb the artist, for how other people see, cr feel, or think, concerns him not at all. In their ordinary life these people, being concerned with their own inner sensations, tend to be reserved and withdrawn from life; they are irresponsive and apathetic. If they have poor self-assertion, they recognize that they are different from others, since they cannot go out to meet life and enjoy it. Further, they are not well organized and integrated, and therefore sufficient unto themselves. For these reasons, they are apt to develop a sense of inferiority, and fall into a neurosis in consequence. If self-assertion is strong, they may break out into fits of rebellion and aggressiveness, which may take a serious asocial direction. Of such stuff the sufferers from Dementia Præcox are made. In these cases the world of phantasy is of the highest importance. Here, all inner sensations have free play to work themselves out and gain full satisfaction, so that this false world becomes more important than the world of reality. Even at the best, however, the introverted sensation type have great difficulty in expressing themselves, and are usually solitary and morose, too often unhappy in their lives, envying the fortunate lot of the easy-going sensational extravert.

The second type, termed by Jung "intuitive," is in some sense the antithesis of the sensation type. The latter is susceptible to impressions, and depends on that part of the complex pattern determining behaviour which arrives so to speak from outside the nervous system, by way of the receptors; the former, on the other hand, depends on that part of the complex, which, it may be said, is within the nervous system in the form of disposition. In other words, intuition is the spontaneous expression of the individual's dispositions or "instincts," using the word in McDougall's sense. As in the sensation type, the discrimination and integrative functions of thought and feeling are poorly developed. They do not control the spontaneous outpouring of the impulses, and this type tends to react in the "all or none" way, glorying in freedom from restraining logical thought. Nor are their feelings in better way, for feeling, organized into sentiments, is also inimical to intuitive expression.

The intuitive is always trying to find an outlet for his

impulses, and the extravert of this type seizes upon objects in the outside world as means to this end. He often perceives association between events which, to others, seem to have little or no connexion, and the future sometimes proves him surprisingly right, but also this same faculty may lead to disaster. The reason for this is, that he approaches these events or objects from a different standpoint from that of any other type. For him, the objects have no value in themselves, but are only important in so far as they can serve the purpose of the development of his own inner impulsion. This gives a quite different associative link from that employed by the sensation type, and so a different outlook results. Once he has used the object, he tends to drop it entirely, since it has no intrinsic value, though at the time he may have regarded it with the greatest enthusiasm. This applies to persons as well as things, and so he appears changeable and fickle. As a rule, he is not a very dependable person, and prefers to wait until the event arrives rather than bind himself by any plans made beforehand. If the inner impulse, which is seeking expression, is in harmony with the needs of the community, he will, in virtue of his new and single approach, see ways out of difficulties which fill the admiring multitude with awe and rapture. But if this impulse runs contrary to the community's needs, then he will appear to throw over his friends or his nation, and almost deliberately lead them astray. Moreover, impulses of value and impulses with no value may succeed one another with bewildering rapidity, and in truth these civic virtues and vices are only incidental, for all that is of importance to the individual is the practical satisfaction of his own inner requirements.

If the intuitive is introverted, he will not be concerned with practical results. He is more interested in how that which comes from within himself, the product of his own engrams, works, and what it leads to, irrespective of outside objects and events. Most of his activity will be in phantasy, and he will be credited with what is called inspiration. The artist, the poet, the prophet, and the mystic are of this class, and, as was the case in the extraverted intuitive, their value depends on whether their inner impulse is in harmony with other needs. If so, then their poetry and their prophecy is hailed as heaven-sent, but if not, then their effusions are regarded as the vague vapourings of an impractical dreamer. As a matter of fact, inasmuch as the engraphic patterns on which the mental activity of this type depends, are the product of long ancestral experience, much of value may be forthcoming, and original points of view may be produced, since their archaic nature is little influenced by consideration of contemporary events. So vivid are the inspirations which arise, that the individual does not always recognize them as products of his own mind. This gives rise not only to hallucinations proper, but to impressions that someone else has told him what to say. This is exemplified by many of the prophets of old, who believed that the voice of God whispered His message in their ear.

Since these four types are the basis of the remaining types, and the latter are no more than higher developments of the same fundamental material, an illustration of how they would be expected to react to a given situation may make for greater clarity. Suppose A is of the extraverted sensation type, B of the introverted sensation type, C of the extraverted intuitional, and D of the introverted intuitional types, how would all these react to an event which must affect them all, such as the announcement of the armistice in November 1918?

A would receive this astounding news, and immediately forget everything else in the overwhelming joy and relief of the moment. If he went out into the crowd, contact with his fellows would lower his general control, and the excess of his feelings would lead him into extravagant and perhaps foolish actions. Of such was Mafeking night.

B would tend to go away by himself and be glad; he might permit himself a private carouse. He would be annoyed by the noisy crowd of A, and retire further afield to be left in peace to think of this new situation, and how it affected him. And then doubt, his old enemy, might creep in. He would ask if it was such a good thing after all? The war was over, with all its opportunities —no more chance of promotion, no possibility now of an M.C. or a D.S.O. If only he had volunteered for that raid, it might have been so different. And so he may work himself up into a very miserable state of mind.

C does not go into the ecstasies of A. To him this presents a new situation. How is he going to use it to his advantage, to the advantage of his inner ambitions, be they towards riches and power, or towards rest and laziness? In either case he applies the event to himself; he must get demobilized at once, and be free; he must buy certain stock, which is sure to go up; whatever it may be, he gets on with the job, in the effort to achieve his end.

D finds this event a new inspiration, his thoughts and feelings may express themselves in a poem of merit, or a mere personal day-dream; unless it be through art, he will not achieve anything practical as a result of the new stimulus, since it has no value either for its own sake, or as an outlet for his impulses, but these may get from it a new turn, so that an original picture or poem is the outcome.

The remaining types described by Jung, which involve the functions of feeling and thinking, represent the attainment of a higher level than those just referred to and, as has been pointed out above, their behaviour corresponds to functions associated with the highest cortical development. Two of these functions are discrimination and integration, and Jung's function of thinking is concerned with discrimination, and that of feeling with integration, at a level at which a considerable measure of syntheses of the lower forms of mental reaction has already been achieved. In either type, the lower levels of sensation or intuition may be recognized as dominant or recessive. In other words, the subject may react chiefly to external impressions, or to inner impulses; but as a rule, these are synthesized into a more or less organized whole. In this way activity depends, not on isolated activations of disparate parts of the total personality, but there is a greater tendency for the whole individual to find expression as a unity. Such synthesis having been achieved, the function of thinking is concerned with discriminating the best method of action, while that of feeling is concerned with organizing the sentiments towards carrying out the required activity. Both of these functions will certainly operate in any individual's mind, for organized activity is impossible without the operation of both the functions of thought and feeling. Yet we say that some people are more addicted to discrimination and thought, and others to integration and feeling leading to action.

The feeling type are those who organize their reactions with external stimuli, or with their inner impulses, as the case may be, so that their personality is dominated by strong emotions, or, if the feeling involved is more prolonged, by moods. These emotions tend to lead to definite actions, carried out to their logical conclusions. A man of this type will feel the need of a great variety of these emotional patterns which enable him to react to the various situations of his life, and he will put great value on these. So much are these feeling reactions important to him, that he will only value those things which are consonant with his feelings, and will reject everything else, but, if his adaptation is good, his feelings will show such great variety and plasticity that there will be few situations which he is not prepared to meet. This is specially so when his attitude is extraverted, for in virtue of this he will be at special pains to adapt himself to outside things and events. He will hedge himself round with organized reactions, which can be called out to meet every conceivable event, and will get on all right until he comes up against the inconceivable event. Then he is at a loss, for having no organization wherewith to meet it, his power of discrimination is recessive and inadequate, and so it is difficult to think out a line of action quickly, to meet the emergency. He will also have a considerable degree of control and understanding, both of his own feelings and those of others. He is never at a loss to recognize what sort of feeling he is experiencing, and will readily discriminate the degree of feeling appropriate to the occasion. He will be able to get into close sympathy with others, and his power of suggestion will be considerable. However, he will necessarily prefer pleasurable feelings to unpleasurable, and may be led from this to try to find things as he wants them to be, and thereby neglect the stern truth and be satisfied with the semblance of things in the form of wish fulfilments. This makes him somewhat unreliable as a scientific observer, for he is apt to twist his facts to fit a priori hypotheses.

As the extravert feeling type wishes to get into harmony with the outside world, so the introvert wishes to get into harmony with himself. He is inwardly sure of himself, but not well adapted to the outside world, and is therefore critical towards it and apt to be criticized by it. This leads to being misunderstood, and to a difficulty of expressing his feeling to others in ordinary social intercourse. Nevertheless, the harmonious integration of his impulses and perceptions may find expression through poetry and art, in the most delicate way, and this type is often deeply religious, having achieved an inner harmony of emotional reactions, organized round a central belief, which becomes all the stronger because the individual is not concerned with, or influenced by the opinions of the outer world, like the extravert of the same type. The best of this type is the real strong silent man who knows what he wants and achieves complete organization of his whole personality towards that end.

If we suppose our hypothetical individuals A, B, C, and D, are organized up to the higher level of the feeling type, we find A receiving and reacting to the joyful news, but never led into the excessive disturbances of "Mafeking" because he can discriminate and control his feelings, both as to their nature and extent. Hence he is never tempted to make a fool of himself, so long as he does not regress from this level, though he may be tolerant and sympathetic to those who do. B is less tolerant of excesses, but is no longer tormented with doubts. He knows and recognizes his own inner feelings, and if, on the whole, he is glad of the cessation of the war, he is filled with an inner content and harmony which he does not trouble to communicate to others. If on the other hand he is disappointed, his very organization of unpleasure may lead him to sink far into melancholy from which it is hard to rouse him.

C, the man of affairs, is still more active and persistent in seizing the opportunity presented, and will probably turn the event to his own great advantage, and if this is in accordance with the requirements of his country, he may be hailed, rather undeservedly, as a great public servant.

D, similarly, has gained strength and sureness by his higher organization, and will be less inclined to lose himself in pure phantasy, and more inclined to rise to a high degree of inspiration in poetry or art. It must be remembered, however, that under the stress of a great emotional stimulus, all may easily regress to the behaviour of the lower types.

As has been said above, the function of thinking is concerned with that of discrimination, knowledge is its province, and classification its business. However, facts are not the only material which serve as the subject of this discrimination; impulses and sensations also come within its purview. The man of the thinking type is concerned with differences, with right and wrong, with this and that, and so has ethics, metaphysics, and much of philosophy for his special field.

The extravert of this type is concerned in his scheme of classification with the objects of outside experience, which he calls facts. Further, he will tend to classify them according to the accepted standards of the community. He will tend to collect an enormous quantity of facts, and cram them into the pigeon-holes already provided for him. When these facts do not quite fit into these pigeon-holes, he is apt to become extremely dogmatic about them, asserting, with no little heat, that they do fit; because they ought to fit! This is so when the type is evolved from a basis of the function of sensation. The chief activity will be directed towards amassing experiences, and these people are good scientific observers, though they may require the corrective of an introvert attitude in properly arranging the facts. If the basis is the function of intuition, the extravert thinker will be interested in the classification of the feelings and impulses of other people, and he will find his interest in history and criticism. He may also achieve eminence in co-ordinating the work of others, as a business organizer. If the extravert thinker is possessed of a narrow outlook, his tendency to force facts into certain accepted categories makes him bitterly hostile to everything which comes outside the limits of these categories, and so he becomes intolerant and bigoted. He is dry, and dull as his feelings are recessive, and, as he cannot pass the bounds of the class in which he places himself, he tends to be a conservative of the die-hard type. The recessive feelings may at times find expression, and if so, they will be uncontrolled and ill-adapted, giving rise to violent outbreaks of temper or other emotional reaction. This is especially liable to be called out in these people if someone does not agree with them, and their rigidity tends to make them carry their theories beyond their legitimate boundaries, so that they insist on a universal applicability; as for example, the ultra-Freudian, who derives every activity from infantile sexuality because he has become impressed with the importance of this latter in certain relationships.

The introvert thinking type moulds the scheme of classification according to lines worked out by himself. If such an individual is of high grade mentality, this is valuable, because the scheme of classification he adopts will be elastic and adaptable. If evolved from a basis of sensation, he will test his observed facts against his scheme, and his scheme against the facts, so that they become adapted to each other. If, however, his mental capacity is less adapted, the scheme of classification he works out may be of little value, and may lead him into the most egregious errors.

If he deals with intuitions, he classifies and criticizes his inner impulses, and in so doing may destroy his usefulness; for he is always considering how and why he does things, and never gets them done. This type of thinker is eminently introspective, and by virtue of the classification of the subjective aspect of experience is more interested in the abstract than the concrete. He more readily understands and sympathizes with other people's faults and difficulties, for he does not classify them according to accepted principles, but recognizes them as subject to the same variations of impulses as he knows so well in himself. For themselves, these individuals are reserved and shy, and do not readily express their opinions. If they do so, they will appear to the extravert, as caring too little for those of others. The opinions of others, indeed, are objective phenomena for which men of the introvert type do not care, but the feelings of others are of much greater subjective interest, and so come more within their purview. Their shyness and reserve make them awkward in company, and the lack of control of their recessive feelings makes their emotional reactions inconsistent and unpredictable. The rules which their subjective function of thought lays down for them lead, however, to the formation of ideals which they often fail to live up to. This induces a feeling of inferiority which they try to compensate by phantasy formation. If this is applied to the ideal of their own character and behaviour, an ever-widening gulf may be formed between reality and phantasy, with disastrous mental conflicts and subsequent neuroses. In any case, this is the type of man who plans before he acts, and who may fail altogether if his plans miscarry, so that in future he never gets beyond the planning stage, lest he should subject himself again to the indignity of failure. However, if his plans succeed, he will often carry out his actions with remarkable persistence and success.

To turn to our cases again, this time organized to exercise the function of thought. A does not join in the crowds of yelling "Mafekers", but he enjoys the fun, stores up all the impressions, and describes them next day with a wealth of enthusiastic detail. He is the journalist actual or potential, with an infinite capacity for receiving and storing impressions, and serving them out again, red-hot from his pen.

B, on the other hand, is interested in the ultimate meaning of all this, the subjective philosophic import. This he may keep to himself, standing aloof, with a somewhat superior air, like Marcus Aurelius, and reflecting on the end of war as a fact and as an ideal. These reflections may or may not be given to the world, according to the degree of introversion, but often they are put down for his private consumption, and the posthumous publication of them by some well-meaning friend must make him turn in his grave.

C is still a man of affairs, but less a man of action than a director of it. He sees how the event may be turned to advantage, but he gets others to carry it out; he is the organizer of the big business, who does not waste himself on details, yet has his finger in every pie. He is helped in this by his capacity for sizing up the impulses and thoughts of others—by his critical and historical capacities, referred to above.

D, as a thinker, is apt to fall into doubt and hesitation again. Discrimination and deliberation play havoc with inspiration; his own impulses are checked by self-criticism, and may die without action being achieved. Still, if his impulses are strong and well organized, he may formulate an ideal and announce to the world his fourteen points. These represent what his own impulses would make of the opportunity, but it is seldom that the acid test of reality permits this dream to come true. This may be fortunate or unfortunate, according as the ideals are noble or fatuous, but he would have to be indeed a superman to achieve a personal ideal of such a sort as to heal all the ills of humanity.

In order to conform with the general scheme of this book, it is necessary to endeavour to examine the physiological implications of this division into types. First of all, from the study of imagery, it is evident that in the case of any individual, activations resulting from certain types of stimulus have more engraphic effect than activations derived from others; or, to put it more colloquially, certain things make a more lasting impression than others. Moreover, amongst the more complex sensory impressions emanating from an object, activation of certain neurones associated with a given sense will be facilitated, as compared to those associated with other senses. For example, let us take as our object "cat", which presents among other patterns of stimuli, cat-picture, cat-sound, cat-smell: and let us take three individuals, A, whose dominant imagery is visual; B, whose dominant imagery is auditory; and C, whose dominant imagery is olfactory. In the case of A, the sight of a cat will immediately bring a visual perception of cat (i.e., attachment of meaning to the sensory impression by association with visual images of similar cats). The sound of a purr, will more slowly bring about perception, and the smell of a cat, perhaps only with difficulty, will imply "cat". Moreover, both purr and smell will induce a visual image of cat, since the engram is so conditioned that there is facilitation of activation of the visual neurones, and relative inhibition of the auditory and olfactory neurones. In an analogous way, B and C will react with greatest ease to auditory and smell stimuli respectively, and will reproduce auditory and olfactory images, with suppression of the other types of imagery. That a dominant imagery involves suppression of other types of imagery and not a complete absence of the latter, is proved by observations, such as those of Rivers who, though entirely deficient in visual imagery in waking life, enjoyed vivid visual images in his dreams. His suggestion that visual imagery is therefore an inferior function, does not seem justified, for the relative facilitation of certain neurones within an engram does not necessarily imply that those which are relatively inhibited are inferior. We see, therefore, that we may divide individuals into various types, according to the nature of their imagery, which in turn depends on the phenomena of facilitation, inhibition and engraphic patterns.

In an analogous way, we can describe the difference between the various types. The extravert, as a whole, is responsive to stimuli coming from without, and this may be due to a relative facilitation of his exteroceptors and their connexions, i.e., the sense organs on the surface of the body, whose function it is to respond to the environment. The introvert, on the other hand, is more responsive to stimuli from within, which may be due to a relative facilitation of his enteroceptors, and their connexions, which, as Sherrington has pointed out, are only secondarily related to the environment. But there is more than this response to specific stimuli in engram activity. We have defined the engram as a pattern of neurones, determined as a more or less definite unit by the mnemic effect of previous activation. Certain engrams are better defined and more specific than others, and the higher the level at which they are integrated, the more complicated is their relatedness, and the less specific they become. Under the circumstances of higher integration, these well-defined engrams are responsive to afferent stimuli from the neurones of another engram as readily, if not more readily than to afferent stimuli from sense organs. Even at low levels, this can be shown to be the case. For example, the desire to micturate and the correlated act, under ordinary circumstances, are induced by a certain degree of tension on the musculature of the bladder, induced by pressure of the urine, and the action is a specific response to this stimulus. However, when the engram which subserves the emotion of intense fear is thrown into activity, the activation may spread to these neurones concerned with the bladder reflex, and produce a similar result to that consequent upon tension of urine on the bladder wall, though this latter normal stimulus may be proved to be absent by clinical observation. Similarly, at higher levels, activation may pass from one engram to another without the intervention of any sensory receptors, whether exteroceptors or enteroceptors, and without obvious glandular or muscular response. It would seem that this activation from one engram to another is more facilitated in the intuitive types than in the sensation types; in other words, in the case of the former the engrams are less specific. So much for the afferent processes. In the activation of the efferent paths there are also differences. In the extravert, activation tends to pass to the neurones of the vegetative system and the motor systems, so that their activity is chiefly in the form of feeling and overt action. In the introvert, the activation tends to pass to those parts of the cortex, such as the frontal lobes and other "silent" areas, which presumably subserve activities less objectively obvious, such as thought. Moreover, other things being equal, direct muscular action will be more commonly observed in either of the empirical types than in the rational types.

The sensation type comprises those in whom the engrams tend to be specifically activated from their receptors, whether exteroceptors or enteroceptors. In the case of the extravert, the response is directly to the environment through the exteroceptors; but in the introvert only indirectly so, through the enteroceptors. Thus Sherrington has described how an exteroceptor receives a stimulus, say of heat, and induces a contraction of a muscle A, but that muscular contraction A stimulates an enteroceptor, which may induce further muscular contracture B. A is a direct response to the environment, but B is a secondary response. This secondary response is characteristic of the introvert sensation type. For example, transfer this process to a higher level, with the necessary complication of the whole reaction, and consider a work of art produced by the extravert and introvert sensation types. Given the reception of the stimulus pattern of a landscape, the first will reproduce a more or less photographic likeness, according to his capacity—a direct response to the environment. The latter may produce a cubist picture, which is his own secondary response to the primary perception.

In the intuitive type, the activation of engrams comes chiefly from a spread from other engrams already established within the nervous system as "instinctive" dispositions, and the distinction between introvert and extravert depends more on the efferent than the afferent phase of the reaction. In the latter, the activity is expressed through feeling and motor activity, i.e., direct motor response; while in the former, it is through thought and phantasy that conation is achieved, that is, by activation of further neurone patterns.

As has been said, the two remaining types involve an organization at a higher level altogether. The function of feeling is concerned with organization, and that of thinking with discrimination. In the feeling type, engrams whose stimulus is derived from the receptors, and others whose stimulus is derived from a spreading of activation from the dispositional engrams, are organized together so as to make for harmony. In the extravert, the engram is so constituted that activations from other engrams are subordinated and fused, so that the responses depending on them are brought into harmony with reactions depending on activation from the receptors. This brings the inner impulses and the total personality into harmony with the outside world. In these cases the major part of the response is dependent on vegetative and motor neurone activity. In the introvert, on the other hand, the complex engram is so organized that the responses, dependent on activation from the receptors are subordinated and fused with the responses dependent on activation resulting from a spread from the dispositional engrams. This results in a harmony of outside impressions and the total personality with the inner impulses. In these the efferent response is mainly through the vegetative and the "silent" areas, and results in emotional religious reflection and artistic expression.

In all the engrams subserving the function of feeling, a large proportion of vegetative neurones are involved, whose activation results in an affective response. In the function of thinking, the engrams involved contain a much smaller proportion of vegetative neurones, and the more abstract the thought that results, the less is the vegetative affective intervention. We know that the cortex possesses the two functions of organization and discrimination, but so far we have no idea by virtue of which neurones these functions are subserved. Therefore, any description of the physiological basis of the two higher functional types must be extremely sketchy at best. For this reason, no more precise indication of the physiological basis of the thinking type can be given than of the feeling type, for the data are the same activation from the receptors in the extravert, and spread from other engrams in the introvert. The difference being, as has already been said, that in the feeling type the function of organization is exercised, while in the thinking type that of discrimination is brought to bear.

In the case of all these types, descriptions have been given of a problematical typical case, but as has been said above, such pure cases are rare, and the recessive or superseded functions will manifest themselves under certain circumstances and on certain occasions. Such alternation of response may lead to considerable general disorganizing and dissociation of the personality, and consequent neurosis. This may be just as true of the higher types as of the lower, for the organization of engrams described by no means involves complete harmony of the mind, though of course it does not preclude an organization of the whole personality, without which mental health is impossible. In the determination and development of the engrams which subserve the various types, the influence of temperament in general, and the relative secretory activity of the endocrine glands in particular, is of the greatest importance and must not be forgotten ; but our knowledge of these factors is so imperfect that no definite suggestions as to their influence can be made, beyond those referred to in Chapter V.

It is obvious that this classification into types is not the only one possible, and others have been attempted by other philosophers ; but there is a value and clarity about Jung's work, which certainly commends itself to those who work among the extremes of these types, whose very departure from the norm, makes it harder for them to adapt to life, and so more liable to fall into neurosis. A follower of Jung, Dr Beatrice Hinkle,[5] worked out a scheme of classification, contemporaneously with the former, which is in many ways similar, but less satisfying. She defines objective, simple, and subjective or bisexual types, of both extravert and introvert attitude, but the choice of the terms objective and subjective are unfortunate, and tend to confuse the issue. However, her treatment of the bisexual type is full of interest and, moreover of great importance, for the recognition of masculine and feminine psychic traits in individuals, irrespective of sex, is a matter of some value, and the conflict between them, in the same individual, merits attention. This matter will, however, be dealt with when Adler's contribution to the study of Personality comes to be discussed in the next chapter.

CHAPTER XI

THE CONTRIBUTION OF ADLER TO THE STUDY OF PERSONALITY

ADLER was the first of Freud's followers who definitely broke away from the school which was founded by the latter. The reason for his defection is obvious, when one comes to consider the divergent philosophic bent of the two men already pointed out in Chapter VIII. The essence of Freud's teaching, as to the "go" of human behaviour, was that the sexual libido drove on the individual by its *vis-a-tergo*, like a leaf before the wind. To this attitude Jung assented to a certain extent, differing on the exact definition of libido, and insisting on the prospective function of man's existence to express something higher. Adler,[1] on the other hand, thought of the end in view of the individual, to gain power and ascendancy over his environment, as the determining factor in moulding human development and behaviour. This prospective view is to a certain extent in accordance with the position adopted in this book, which is based on Alexander's scheme of emergent evolution, with the quality of Deity at the top, the whole cosmos evolving according to certain laws towards this end. It must at once be admitted, however, that the term "end in view" ought not to be used in connexion with an evolutionary scheme, as it may be criticized immediately by asking "end in view of whom or what"? Still, although this term is inaccurate, it is perhaps more permissible, if we accept Lloyd Morgan's[2] concept of Causality—the Deity, who is the immanent law according to which the process of evolution gets itself evolved.* The term end in view is used here however, because it is desired to establish the analogy with Adler's

* Cf. Adler's "Durch das grosse Sein das uns umgibt und weit in uns hineinreicht, zicht sich ein grosses Werden das dem vollendeten Sein zustrebt" ("Through the great Being which surrounds and penetrates us there is a great becoming, which strives toward a completed being").

contention, that in human conduct there is a positing of a final purpose, which determines conduct. So far as this involves the relatedness which we call consciousness, with its characteristic function of prevision, the term "end in view" is not amiss, but the process may go on at levels lower than those which involve consciousness, and consequently it must be used with caution. Adler also disagrees with Freud in the latter's contention that the sex impulse is the basis of all neurotic, and much of normal behaviour. For Adler, sexual aberrations, both in reality and phantasy, are but symbolic manifestations of the striving of the ego to reach the final goal of complete masculinity, which involves sexual dominance, and which, at any rate in the neurotic, is the goal, which is always desired and never reached, This concept of the striving towards the complete man is very similar to the will to power of Nietzsche, and involves a heightening of the ego ideal and the ego consciousness. Adler's work is of course based on a study of the neuroses, but the behaviour of the neurotic is a crude and sometimes debased caricature of that of the normal man, and so is of service in the study of personality as a whole, as has been said before. Moreover Adler's original approach to the study of the neurotic constitution was from the organic and temperamental standpoint. This approach is all too rare, and for this reason, if for no other, his work demands consideration. He started from a conception of what he calls organ inferiorities and their compensations. Thus, it is a commonplace of pathology that if one organ such as the kidney is congenitally deficient, it is found that the other shows compensatory hypertrophy. Similarly, in the endocrine system, deficiencies of one gland are often met by a compensatory hypertrophy of other glands of the same group. Such are examples of physical compensations for physical deficiencies. Nor does this compensatory activity always result harmoniously for the individual, for many cases of hyperthyroidism seem to depend on this attempt at compensation for deficiency in other glands. Adler contends that correlated with the physical inferiority, there is at the same time a psychic inferiority, and *pari passu* a psychic compensatory activity. This compensatory activity he calls the will to power. There is a certain difference between the ways in which this will to power is manifested, and this will depend, amongst other things, on the organ which is, or which is thought to be inferior. But Adler holds that in almost all cases of inferiority of bodily organs there is an inferiority of the sexual apparatus. This accounts for the frequency of the sexual element in the psychic compensation. That inferiorities in the sexual apparatus are apt to accompany inferiorities elsewhere, is borne out by Mott's[3] work on Dementia Præcox. He found out that, along with degenerative changes in the Betz cells of the cortex, i.e., the highest type of nerve cell, there were changes in the testicular cells. Neither of these degenerations were the cause or effect of the other, but simply coincident phenomena.

The compensation may or may not be successful. The classical example of successful compensation is Demosthenes the stammerer, who became the greatest orator of Greece, his particular career being probably determined by the specially inferior organ. If we can accept the evidence that Julius Cæsar and Napoleon were epileptics, they may also be taken as successful psychic compensations of organ inferiority, along the lines of the Will to Power, though the typical egocentric ruthless mentality of the epileptic also contributed to their characters. Adler does not infer that complete Masculinity or the Nietzschen Superman is the goal of every individual, but only of those whose psychic appreciation of inferiority leads to a constant comparison between themselves and those around them, generally to the detriment of themselves. Such comparisons restrict the attention to the opposition of the ego to the environment, instead of to the harmony of the ego with the environment. The result is the dominance of a narrow self-regarding sentiment, which may result in the overriding of all opposition and the material success of the individual. If, however, this sentiment is not well organized, and is in opposition to the environment, the compensation will be inadequate, and neurosis or other abnormal behaviour will result almost inevitably. It would appear, therefore, that Adler's contributions to psychology are only applicable in full to those whose self-regarding sentiment has, in Janet's phrase, a small radius of action. Yet, there is probably no one in whom the sense of inferiority is absent, and who does not indulge in the correlated attempts at compensation which lead to an aggressiveness merely masking the former. In other words, there is no one who has achieved perfect harmony with the environment, and who does not find himself in opposition to his surroundings, from time to time. In passing, this throws additional doubt on the correctness of McDougall's treatment of self-assertion and self-abasement as primary instinctive dispositions, without more careful discrimination of their incidence. May they not be secondary reactions to organ inferiorities, which are definitely established as the result of experience and contact with the environment? Those individuals who succeed in achieving, even approximately, full compensation for their inferiorities are few. We cannot all attain the level of Demosthenes or Napoleon, and, on the whole, it is probably a good thing for the world, that we cannot. As has been said, many people have a self-regarding sentiment, of narrow radius, but of close organization. The neurone pattern which subserves this sentiment is so engraphically conditioned that spread of activation from engrams, subserving behaviour opposed to the function of this sentiment, is inhibited; while activation from those subserving behaviour in accordance with its object is facilitated. In the majority of people there is a certain degree of failure in the effort of compensation, and this necessarily leads to a want of coincidence, between ideals and achievement. This divergence is apt to become progressively wider. The more the individual realizes his incapacity for action, the higher is he apt to put his ideals. He is constantly saying to himself, "If only I could do this, how splendid it would be!" and as he does not get it done, he raises the ideal to the highest possible level, so as to excuse himself for his failure. For if he does this, he can always satisfy himself that the task which is set him is too difficult, and at the same time reassure himself by the reflection that if he could only accomplish it, he would be so very superior to his fellows. This however, reacts to his detriment; for with every failure he gets still more discouraged, and so the gulf continues to widen. Such a state of affairs leads to all sorts of consequences in conduct. The individual tends to do less and less, and leaves undone many things which are well within his capacity. The more he feels his incapacity, the less he does, and so he starts to put things off, to excuse himself and to shirk. Carried to extremes, this shirking amounts to a deadly sin. It results in a search for means to avoid doing those things which are the individual's chief duty, and the logical consequence is that he strives to find a situation in which others shall take on all responsibility, or where all his own duties shall cease. The former may lead to an enslavement of some unfortunate relative, parent, child, husband or wife, as the case may be, who shall decide everything, and ultimately do everything, while the neurotic—for at this level he is assuredly a neurotic—sits and whines about what he would like to be doing if only he were not so afflicted. Or his desire to place his responsibilities on others may take a more general form, and he may play with the idea of insanity. For this means that he will no longer be held responsible for his actions, and will be cared for by others. The phantasy of going insane then becomes a wish fulfilment. However, the idea of life in an asylum is not in harmony with many of his other sentiments, and, as it gives rise to a feeling of dread, there is a conditioning of the wish to be protected and cared for in an institution, with the fear of what it involves. The patient feels that a frank wish for insanity is not in accordance with his ego-ideal, and so this idea never appears in consciousness as a wish, but always as a fear, the conditioned feeling being dominant. To wish for insanity is a disgrace, but to fear insanity is reputable, and therefore possible. Similarly, the wish that responsibility should end altogether has its logical outcome in the idea of suicide. Again, there is a conditioning with fear which is usually so strong that there is not the slightest chance of suicide being actually carried out. The unfortunate individual merely plays with these ideas, which are really temptations analogous to that of taking money, or any such criminal offence; and it frequently happens that if the subject can be got to recognize this, their true significance, he has taken the first step towards recovery. So much for the attitude of the individual with the sense of inferiority towards himself. With regard to others, he will first envy those who can do better than he can. From this he will protect himself with the idea that he is specially unfortunate, whether in his social position, in his upbringing, and more particularly, in his state of health. Later he will begin to disparage the character and work of his neighbour, which is merely another way of defending himself from the consciousness of his own inferiority. Next, there will be a tendency to try to get the better of his rivals by foul means, if not by fair. This reaction is an extremely common one in determining the delinquencies of children, as will be seen in Chapter XIV. It is not suggested that there is no other explanation of selfish and evil behaviour than that of organ inferiority and its psychic compensation, for dispositional and environmental conditions play their part. However, there is no doubt that this temperamental factor in the determining of behaviour is important and that the sense of inferiority and the will to power, are very common, and have a great deal to do with such types of behaviour. A concrete example may serve to illustrate, how these reactions may affect a person's life. A girl had a curvature of the spine, of which she became extremely conscious at an early age. She very soon got a definite sense of inferiority in relation to her school fellows, and from this developed an intense will to power. At first, it manifested itself in the practice of running down to school, so that she arrived before other children living in the same district as herself. She thus proved to herself that she was quite as good, if not better than the others, so far as fleetness of foot was concerned. It then spread to games, and she strove to excel in all sorts of ways which were really beyond her strength. If anybody beat her, she felt intensely jealous, and did not rest until she had overcome her rival in some direction or other, to make up for her defeat. With her work it was the same thing. This went on until she really overtaxed her strength, and became ill. An unfortunate diagnosis of heart disease gave her an excuse which she used all through life. Whenever she was called upon to do anything which was beyond her strength, or rather her own estimation of her strength, she had an attack of palpitation which was really induced by the auto-suggestion that it would be convenient to have palpitation, and a fear lest her inferiority should prevent her accomplishing the task. A love affair, which turned out badly, completed her sense of inferiority. From this time she became really inefficient and neurotic. Her heart was always bothering her. Yet she was unwilling to admit that anybody could manage things in her home, but herself. She would have spurts of energy in which she would do a tremendous lot, at a great pace, only to collapse in the middle, and leave others to clear up the mess. Such behaviour was always put down to her unfortunate illness; and the short intervals of energy went to prove her tremendous keenness to work hard, if she only could. This explanation gave considerable satisfaction to herself, though it was not received at quite the same valuation by her relatives. Needless to say, she herself was not happy, she felt misunderstood, no doctor ever realized "how ill" she was, or could cure her complaint. When eventually an attempt was made to show her the real truth, she resented this intensely, and went off elsewhere, preferring to keep up the fiction of physical disease, rather than face the difficulties of life. She still kept up the childish habit of trying to walk faster than others, and was on the lookout as to how she could get the better of other people in small things. She was inclined to envy and malice, but held it as a decided grievance, that she was not popular. This increased her feeling of being misunderstood, and with it her self-pity, and so things went on from bad to worse.

As has been said, Adler holds that the final goal of both sexes is complete masculinity, and the inference is that this is never attained. The antithesis to masculinity is femininity, and it can never be too strongly insisted that in any individual there is an admixture of both these characteristics. Psychically, at any rate, man is bisexual, and this is borne out in the field of physical structure by anatomical modifications; for in the most normal males there is a vestige of the female genital organs, in the prostatic utricle; and similarly in the female, the clitoris is the analogue of the penis. Nor is it by any means uncommon to find more marked abnormalities, in the form of female sex characteristics occurring in the male, and vice versa. This anomaly occasionally reaches the stage of true hermaphroditism, where the determination of sex becomes a matter of difficulty. In relation to the question of psychic correlations, it is held by many authorities that the true homosexual of either sex has always a considerable degree of over-development of the physical characters of the opposite sex. That this is not universally true of obvious sex characters is certain, but it would be of interest to know whether a microscopical examination of testis or ovary, as the case might be, would reveal tissue properly belonging to the opposite sex. However, such anatomical researches have not been carried out on a sufficiently large scale to give reliable evidence. Nevertheless, recent experiments have shown the interchangeability of sex characteristics, both physical and psychical. Crew[4] described how a hen took on certain physical and behaviouristic characters of the cock, after destruction of the ovaries by tubercular disease. Tolman[5] has described experiments in which ovarian tissue was grafted into castrated rats, with the result that the quondam male took on the functions of nest building, and mothering the young. Conversely, testicular tissue was grafted into ovariectomized rats, with the result that the quondam female went through all the copulatory movements characteristic of the male. These facts prove that there is, even on the physical side, no such hard and fast differentiation into the male and the female as at first sight seems probable, and it is certain that on the psychical side this is even more evident. That this is so may be judged by the difficulties which beset us when we try to formulate the typical psychical characteristics of male and female. Adler holds that complete masculinity is the goal, not only of the male but also of the female, and there is a good deal to be said for it in the neurotic, but it is not so in the normal individual. As Hinkle[6] has pointed out, woman has a very definite function, and there is no justification in supposing that the normal woman desires any other development than that of her own biological function. On the other hand, she does have certain masculine traits within her, and recent social developments have permitted these more free development. Hence we find that some apparently normal women, who have fulfilled their normal biological function, do break down, because these masculine ego impulses have found no outlet.

One of the characteristic features of the human race, as opposed to the animals, is that the former have to a certain extent translated the sexual impulse so that it no longer serves a strictly biological function but serves the pleasure of the ego. This is in accordance with the continuity of the period of active desire in man, as compared to the œstral cycle in animals. Although this applies to both sexes, there is little doubt that women have retained a much closer touch to the biological creative impulse, which was the original function of the sex pattern. Man on the other hand, although he may owe such tendency to create, as he possesses, to the feminine attributes in his make-up, translates his creation to the sphere of thought or manipulation, thereby becoming an artist, and no man is without any artistic capabilities. In both the artist and the woman, the tendency is to sacrifice the self-preservation, or ego impulses, to the created being, be it child or work of art, whereas the more normal man tends to sacrifice his sexual and creative impulses to his ego, and to his individual purposes. The identification of the artist and the woman in their creative orientation is, to a certain extent, borne out by the other features of their personality, for not only are many artists feminine in type, but even those who are masculine show a consciousness of a delicacy and sensitiveness which is more characteristic of the woman than of the man. For example Maeder[7] describes, how the Swiss artist Hodler, who was of the dominant masculine type, bewailed the fact that no one would recognize and give him credit for the woman that was in him. For women therefore, these creative impulses are essentially biological, real, and practical, hence her tendency to be interested chiefly in people and things. For man the creative impulses are no longer biological, and can be translated to phantasy and theory. Hence he is free to experiment, and to enquire into the whys and wherefores, to seek to propound the laws which govern himself and nature. If we refer back to the fundamental impulses of self-preservation and race-preservation, it would appear that, on the whole, the man's emotional dispositions tend to be integrated in relation to the former, while the woman's are integrated in relation to the latter. For example, the emotion of anger is felt more strongly by the man in relation to himself, his career, and his own concerns with the environment, whereas the woman feels this emotion more strongly in relation to her sexual life and her offspring. The same is true of curiosity, and to a certain extent of fear. This leads to the development of the ego in relation to the environment being the dominant interest in the average man, so that his career and his own progress through life become of the first importance. Such a result is only partially due to biological factors, for the demands of social life and civilization have done much to promote this orientation. With the woman, on the other hand, the dominant interest is with the sexual life in the broadest sense of the term, with home, husband

and children, as her chief concern. Moreover, she is essentially biologically creative and this creation is the centre of her emotional life. Bloch[8] declares that man is more aggressive, progressive, and variable, while woman is more submissive, receptive, and suggestible. Adler attributes to the masculine ideal certainty, superiority and self-esteem, i.e. a place in the sun, but this seems a one-sided view, vitiated by the fact that he is discussing neurotics who, according to him, always aim at a masculine ideal, turning altogether aside from any possible feminine ideal. Attempts at exact definition as to what constitutes the psychic constitution of the woman as opposed to the man have been unsatisfactory, since it was first attempted by Havelock Ellis[9] in his *Men and Women*, which enumerated a mass of statistical variations between the sexes, without arriving at any composite picture that seemed to fit the individual man or woman. That this is so, is undoubtedly due to the fact that as in the physical sphere, so in the psychic sphere, there are always recessive vestiges of the opposite sex which confuse the analysis of the personality, and when there is any considerable prominence of the recessive characters, a state of conflict is readily induced. In this respect there is a lot of sense in the remark of the Theosophist lady, in Nicholson's *Marriage Craft*, who described the ideal of harmonious marriage as the wedding of the masculine and feminine traits in one individual. Hinckle has discussed these contrasting characteristics in relation to her classification into types, referred to in the last chapter. She describes the masculine and feminine symbols respectively as follows:—"The father" (the male symbol) "stands for the demand of reality to face the world and to take one's place in the outer life of effort and struggle. It is the dominant aggressive factor in phantasy, the symbol of power, of domination and authority, of practical life in the world, and signifies the individual and ego side of the personality." "The mother" (the female symbol), "on the other hand, is the typical symbol of love, of understanding, of care, of compassion and tenderness, the mediation between the child and the world, or the father; the original spring, out of which altruism has developed. She is the one who softens the path, on whom the child can depend and rely in need, and represents the protecting, collecting and feeling side of human personality." The conflict between these two orientations in any individual unquestionably gives rise to trouble, and in many women there is an effort to attain to the masculine orientation, which only occasionally meets with success, and when it fails, neurosis is apt to ensue. It is suggested, that in certain men there is a tendency to seek the feminine orientation, but the success of this attainment of the opposite, is even less probable in man than in woman. For it is more against all social convention that a man should be feminine, than that a woman should be masculine, especially during the last 25 years. Hence, in the case of the effeminate man, there is apt to be a secondary superficial swing in the opposite direction, with what Adler calls an exaggerated masculine protest, which may disguise the deeper impulse towards femininity. As has been said, it is not known to what extent these divergencies towards the opposite sex depend on physical temperamental influences; but experiments, such as those quoted of Crew and Tolman, make it seem probable that anomalies in sex gland differentiation may play an important part. The bisexual manifestations may exhibit themselves in various ways. In the man, there may be a definite tendency to homosexuality, the rôle in such cases being as a rule passive, though the complication induced by the reaction of the masculine protest may determine an active rôle, though maintaining the homosexual object. Similarly, there may be masochistic manifestations, with secondary sadistic tendencies, dependent on the protest reaction. Or there may be normal orientation of sexual desire; but in his emotional reactions to both sexes, the man may show a submissive, clinging, rather sentimental attitude, which is more characteristic of a woman than of a man. He may be of the "domestic" type, who is continually concerning himself with details of the home and children, the type women are apt to find meddlesome and in the way, and from whom they would gladly welcome a little wholesome neglect. In the intellectual sphere, it is more difficult to describe the characteristics, for the difference between man and woman is more obscure, but the feminine man will be concerned to a greater extent than usual with facts of immediate interest, which he may accumulate in his memory without much concern for their relative significance, or practical utility, since he is not really in such fundamentally close touch with things as they really are, as is the woman. Similarly, in the woman of this reversed type there may be a secondary reversion to the feminine ideal, often induced by the dictates of society, but as a rule this is not so strong as in the case of the man, and the conflict is usually between genuine feminine characteristics, and genuine masculine traits, so that her conduct may at one time appear as being almost aggressively feminine, while at another she exhibits behaviour which would be more natural in a man. Like her counterpart of the other sex, she may show actual homosexual tendencies, and as a rule the tendency will be to adopt the active rôle. Similarly, she may show sadistic impulses, in accordance with her general aggressiveness. The orientation of her sexual desire may be normal, however, but in the emotional sphere she may tend to be aggressive and independent. Such a woman wishes to go out in the world and carve out a career for herself; she often chooses for her husband a man of the type described above, and becomes the dominant partner in the ménage, and moreover, given sufficient general capacity, runs the establishment remarkably well. In the intellectual sphere, she is interested in more abstract questions than is usually the case with women. She will be concerned with the hows and whys, and readily discriminates the relative values of her experience. Types such as have been described are, of course, somewhat extreme, but the tendency to make for the opposite ideal is never absent and the "complete man" and the "complete woman" do not really exist.

In dealing with the psychological differences between the sexes, in addition to the influence of the secretions of the gonads, the tertiary psychic factors arising from a consciousness of belonging to one or other sex must be remembered. Evidence has already been adduced to show that secondary female characteristics are grafted on to the more primary male characters, rather than the other way about. Studies of children and certain psycho-analytical investigations have further shown that modesty and passivity which are essentially characteristic of the female, are not primarily given in the female child, but that they are induced through a somewhat prolonged course of development, under the dictates of environmental and bodily influences, from a primary aggressive active attitude, comparable to that of the male.

The passivity which is characteristic of the female is of

considerable interest, for as Brierley[10] points out, the ego impulse of all individuals, both male and female, is active and katabolic. In the male, the sex impulse is also active and katabolic, so that there is no special conflict between sex and ego, and they may continue on parallel courses. In the female, however, the sex impulse is more passive and anabolic, so that it is in opposition to the ego, and somehow or other they have to find a compromise. This compromise is afforded by marriage and maternity in many cases, and a relative stability is established by the biological creativity of the rearing of children, but in certain married women, whose ego impulse dominates the sex impulse, and in unmarried women in whom the compromise has not been achieved, there is apt to be a marked instability, which tends to neurosis. Even in these women whose ego is so dominant that they succeed in repressing sex, and establish successful careers for themselves, it too often happens that the repression is only successful for a time, and that later in life they break down and become neurotic. In those women in whom the compromise has been successful, however, there is necessarily a firm organization of the ego and sex impulses to one end, and this organization limits the variation in type of women, as compared to man, so that they do tend to conform to an average.

In all the attempts to differentiate intellectual differences between the sexes, it is shown that there is no one point in which males as males excel, or females as females excel; but what does come out in these studies is that there is much more individual variation in boys than there is in girls. This closer approximation to the average in the case of the female is noticeable in many aspects of life. She tends to be rather more conventional—to pay more attention to fashions and public opinion. In the male, the ego impulse and the sex impulse run parallel, but are not necessarily organized together, so that a man may keep his career perfectly distinct from his home life, in a way that a woman finds hard to understand. Similarly, the various components of his sentiment of love are less closely organized, so that he can more readily separate the physical component from the rest, without a complete disorganization of the sentiment, or transference of its object, than is the case in the majority of women. Obviously, such remarks only apply to general tendencies, and there will be plenty of individual exceptions. How far the recent "emancipation" of women has tended to obliterate these differences is an interesting study, though out of place here, but the suggestion conveyed by modern manners is that "feminine" behaviour is more due to the influence of the community than to inherent differences, which is in accordance with Crew's biological finding, that when femininity decays masculine characteristics become unmasked.

To sum up these observations, every individual is a combination of masculine and feminine characteristics, one or other of which preponderates, usually, but not always in accordance with the manifest sex. Masculinity is associated with the self-preservation group in the disposition and the aggrandizement of the ego, and is manifested by physical strength and emotional self-assertion, while intellectually the interest is given to generalizations and principles of action. Femininity is associated with the race-preservation group in the disposition, and the creation of something outside the self. It is manifested physically, by grace and delicacy of manipulation, emotionally by submissiveness, which may rise to self-sacrifice, and intellectually the interest is focused on objects and actual action. The normal man pursues the ideal of masculinity with a greater or less degree of success. The normal woman pursues the ideal of femininity with a more or less happy issue. The male may be so constituted as to pursue a feminine ideal, in which case he is artistic in some way or other, and generally unbalanced and even neurotic. Similarly the female may (Adler would say does) pursue a masculine ideal, in which case she will usually, sooner or later, develop neurosis.

In the study of Personality, the contribution of Adler merits careful attention, especially in respect of his temperamental approach to the problem. His concept of compensations for inferiorities, both in the physical and psychical fields, are of almost universal application, and although the goal of complete masculinity does not seem to hold good in every case, it throws much light on the difficult question of psychical sex differentiation. In the latter case the "drive to the opposite" does not seem to be a compensation for inferiority, unless it be an inferiority to harbour germ plasm, properly belonging to the other sex, but rather a reaction determined by temperamental factors, which run counter to the general "go" of the bodily influences. In other words, in spite of a general "end in view" it seems reasonable to agree with Freud, that it is the inherent constitution which is responsible for development, whether in respect of bodily structure or of behaviour But whether the will to power be considered as a striving towards such an end, or an effort to overcome inherent obstacles, there can be no denying its existence in every individual. Moreover, the greater the inherent sense of inferiority, the greater may be the will to power; indeed, without this conflicting duality the sum of human achievement would be vastly lessened. But every man has his Achilles heel somewhere, and to Adler must be given the credit for working this out scientifically. We know as a result of this work, that the strong ambitious man has somewhere or other a weak spot in his armour, an inferiority which is often hidden even from himself. He may get through life without discovery, but it is remarkable how often the arrows of fate find and wound the "heel," wherever it may be.

CHAPTER XII

THE CONTRIBUTION OF KEMPF TO THE STUDY OF PERSONALITY

THE work of Kempf[1] throws an interesting sidelight on psycho-analytic theory in relation to Personality. An ardent behaviourist, and a convinced believer in Freud's doctrines, he attempts to find a physiological basis for his conclusions. He advances the thesis, that all overt behaviour is the direct result of the alterations in tension of autonomic segments. Under the term autonomic segments, he includes all the vegetative systems of the body, circulatory, respiratory, digestive, urinary, and genital; all the endocrine glands, and the vegetative nervous system, both sympathetic and autonomic. The various "segments," digestive, circulatory, genital and the like, are subject to "affective cravings," involving changes in the postural tensions of their musculature. By the postural tension, or tone of a muscle, is meant the degree of static contraction of that muscle, which is necessary, in conjunction with other muscles in a similar state of static contraction, to maintain the limb or the organ in its ordinary position of rest. Thus, the hand at rest usually maintains a position with the fingers semi-flexed. To retain this posture, both flexors and extensors must maintain a certain degree of contraction. This static contraction is the postural tone. Sherrington[2] demonstrated the existence of the postural tone of muscles, both striped and unstriped, and this varies with the variation in affective states. Thus, it is known that in the case of the stomach, hunger is accompanied by changes in the postural tension, amounting to definite contractions. Kempf maintains that these contractions are the direct cause of hunger, or in other words, that hunger is the perception of kinesthetic impulses arising from the change in postural tone of the stomach. Such changes of tension in the various autonomic segments represent a demand for satisfaction of the biological needs of an animal, for the maintenance of the life of the individual on the one hand, and continuance of the race on the other. But, with the advance of complexity in the animal organism, it became necessary, if these needs were to be fulfilled, for the animal to shift itself about in the environment, in order to find the means of satisfaction. Hence, in the course of biological evolution it became requisite for the continuance of animal species that a "projicient system" should be developed. This consists of the central nervous system and muscular apparatus. To refer once more to the illustration afforded by the alterations of postural tone in the stomach which are accompanied by hunger, we have here a demand for satisfaction of an organic need. This demand corresponds to the Freudian "wish." The "wish" or state of tension has an unpleasant affective value. According to the "pleasure principle," this tension must be relieved, and the organism must find means to do so. These means can only be attained by interaction of organism with the environment, and by the establishment of two new apparati. Firstly, there must be established appropriate receptor patterns to respond to the stimuli representative of the wish for satisfaction, that is to say, in the case of hunger—suitable food. This receptor pattern, will be composed of an associated complex of sensory nerve endings, comprised in the various exteroceptive sense organs, whereby the appropriate food can be smelt, tasted, touched, seen, etc. Secondly, a correlated mechanism must be evolved whereby the food, from which these stimuli originate, may be approached and ingested. In addition, for the better furtherance of this object, it may be necessary to move the animal about in space so that the receptor pattern may be brought in contact with the suitable stimuli, and not merely left to respond if the said stimuli arrive in the neighbourhood. This may involve an active voluntary search for edibles, in the case of hunger, or for a mate, in the case of sexual cravings. An example may illustrate the sequence of events as follows. Certain alterations in postural tone of the stomach arise in response to metabolic requirements of certain fluids and solids. As the result of the kinesthetic impulses so aroused, hunger is experienced. The "affective craving" hunger facilitates certain receptors and their connexions, which respond to the various properties, colour, shape and odour of the orange which is lying on a neighbouring table. This combined with memory images of taste, and the general mass of experience relating to orange, leads to the perception—orange, and further perhaps to the judgment—good to eat. Or the process may become more complicated if there is no orange or other food handy, and it becomes necessary to take some money from a drawer, go out of the house, and proceed to a shop and buy one. Once the orange has been acquired, certain muscular movements are brought into play, whereby the orange is seized, peeled and conveyed to the mouth, and so reaching the stomach, allays the hypertension. Thus the cycle is completed, the wish is fulfilled, pleasure is attained, and a state of quiescence ensues. Similar cycles may be traced from conditions of hypertension (appetitive), or hypotension (aversive), in the other autonomic segments, and do not require further elaboration. As may naturally be expected from a psycho-analytic enthusiast, the hypertension and hypotensions of the genital segment are held to influence behaviour in an overwhelming proportion of cases. The study of pathological personalities bears this out to a very great extent, and there can be no question that the same applies to more of the behaviour of normal individuals than many are willing to admit, for the tensions in the complicated patterns associated with sex do vary both frequently and violently. But the sex impulses become so commingled with other impulses in the composition of the personality, and in so doing there emerge such totally different and distinct qualities, that to analyse these behaviours and qualities to the level where the sex impulse entered into their composition, no more explains them, than hydrogen and oxygen explain water. We may, if we like, say that a diamond is nothing but carbon, and we may say that chivalry is nothing but an attempt to satisfy the affective craving of the genital segment, but such statements explain neither the one nor the other, for with a new relatedness, a new quality emerges. Kempf indeed gets over the difficulty of the modification of his primary affective cravings, by reference to the process of conditioning. Basing his arguments on this well-known process in physiology, demonstrated by Pawlow and others, he shows how the primary affective cravings are constantly met with resistances from the environment. The struggle between these resistances and the affective cravings leads to increasing efforts to control the environment. This necessitates the increase in skill, self-knowledge and self-control, and *pari passu*, the increase in complexity of the projicient system. At first the affective cravings demand response to specific stimuli directly ministering to their needs, but in view of the conflicting interests, and demands of the different autonomic segments, and to the resistances opposed by the environment, they soon begin to seek quite a different set of stimuli, in response to which they more or less succeed in achieving mutual satisfaction. The conditioning process, therefore, leads to the development of new receptor patterns and new behaviour patterns, so that the apparent end in view may be very different from that which would subserve the direct satisfaction of the original affective craving. This leads to the process of sublimation, whereby the various needs of the individual are modified so as not to oppose each other, or the demands of the community. Where the process of conditioning does not proceed smoothly, the processes of repression, suppression, regression and the rest, arise. He lays particular stress on the influence of the family in conditioning the affective cravings of the young child. In Kempf's work, the conflict between the youth striving for emancipation, and age striving to maintain authority, is exemplified by a wealth of detail, both from mythology and literature and real life. In fact, from this point, Kempf follows the general trend of psycho-analytic doctrine, and reference to this does not need to be repeated here. In discussing the personality, Kempf insists on the conception of a unity which, in the light of the concept of emergence, is insisted on here. The development of such personality involves the sublimation of affective cravings and the correlation of projicient reactions. "From birth the autonomic apparatus, having been forced to abandon its parasitical attachment to the mother, begins its struggle of co-ordinating its projicient apparatus into an efficient instrument, with progressive refinements of self-control and skill of adaptation, in order to keep up with the standards of its rivals and the race. Upon the nature of the skilful co-ordination, and the conditioning of the cravings, depends the existence of the biological potency (of social influence and fitness, commercial and sexual prowess, and sexual potency)". The object of this sublimation and correlation, he describes as the pursuit of goodness and happiness, which can only be obtained by a free outlet, whereby the demands of autonomic cravings can be met, when suitably modified to avoid friction with the requirements of the environment. To achieve this goal, it is necessary that the individual should at once be adaptable and correlated, and that the requirements of the environment should not be too insistent and hard to surmount. There can be no question that in modern civilized society there is a tendency for the requirements of the environment to present too great an obstacle for all but the best and strongest personalities. If the personality is going to succeed in reacting to the environment, it must act as a unity. All the segmental affective cravings must react in a correlated way, otherwise dissociation takes place, and the possibility of adaptation ceases. If the dictates of society repress the proper development of any one of these affective cravings, then the whole personality becomes lop-sided, and a neurosis of some sort is apt to occur. The most common mental conflict in the individual is that between the demands of these affective cravings, and the effort to retain the approval and esteem of the family, or of society in general. In the normal healthy individual a working compromise is reached ; in the neurotic, the affective craving is repressed, and an effort is made to retain the esteem of society and the self, at the expense of a craving which will not be denied. This leads to the inner dissociation, which brings the individual up against himself; the state of mind so characteristic of the neurotic. When the desire to retain social esteem is repressed, then the affective cravings are allowed full play, and a conflict arises between the ego and the community. For the ego, this means asocial delinquency; for the community, an enemy who must be suppressed.

This brief exposition may give some conception of the thesis advanced by Kempf, and there is no doubt that it is one which is attractive from its very simplicity. He admits, that although the autonomic segments are the prime movers in determining behaviour, with the development of the projicient apparatus, they are in turn controlled and modified by the more elaborate system. There can be no question that these affective cravings determine much in behaviour, and that many reactions are the resultants of kinesthetic and other stimuli arising within our bodily organs. Indeed, there seems a risk of neglecting the enormous importance of these inner stimuli as initiators of behaviour, to which the work of Kempf is a wholesome corrective. But to suggest that all behaviour, which is a sequel of the stimuli arriving from outside of the body, is only so in virtue of pre-existing autonomic cravings, seems carrying matters too far. Further, it would imply that the vegetative nervous system is phylogenetically and ontogenetically older than the projicient nervous system, since, according to Kempf, the latter is only evolved to meet the demands of the former. For this there does not seem to be sufficient evidence. Embryological studies show that the cells of the vegetative nervous system are derived from the neural crest, and in part, from the neural tube, and are not, as was at one time supposed, of separate mesoblastic origin. It is definitely stated in the last edition of Cunningham's *Anatomy*, that "The sympathetic nervous system is essentially dependent on, and subservient to, the central nervous system, from which it can be no more separated sharply, either anatomically or developmentally, than can the rest of the peripheral nervous system." Similarly, zoological findings show that there is no particular reason to differentiate the very primitive nervous system of the Cœlenterates, as either vegetative or projicient; while in the Vermes, the zoologist already distinguishes certain ganglia as sympathetic, which are clearly developed from the skeletal segmental or central ganglia.[3] On these grounds, it seems difficult to see why the central nervous system should be supposed to have developed as a response to the demands of the autonomic cravings for satisfaction. Such a doctrine would suggest that animal life was evolved from plant life, whereas they are separate evolutionary developments, arising with the emergence of life.

Again, the acceptance of the doctrine of Kempf as the complete explanation of all behaviour, involves the whole-hearted acceptance of the James-Lange theory of emotion, that the emotions, as felt, are nothing but the kinesthetic impressions, originating from the alteration of postural tensions in unstriped muscle. As McDougall[4] points out, this implies that before an emotion is felt these bodily changes in tension must take place, but this is as manifestly untrue as to say that to experience the image of an orange, the retina and the taste buds must be stimulated.

Imagery of the sensations which go to make up emotion, is as possible as images of sight and taste. A more important objection however, pointed out by McDougall, is that this theory leaves out of account the conative impulse to act which is inherent in the organization of the patterns of nerve cells that are activated in response to stimuli, and which is an essential part of an emotion. Kempf does not of course deny this conative impulse, but does not give it a place inherent in the organization of an emotional pattern, and postulates the intervention of the bodily tensions before it can be activated. It would seem that emotion is an emergent from a much more complex pattern than these views would suggest. Mosso,[5] in his experiments on the contracting bladder, has shown the influence of the sympathetic nervous system in relation to emotional expression, but he does not prove that the muscular activity resulting from sympathetic activity, precedes the psychic response to the stimulus. Cannon[6] has shown how the internal secretions play a part; how for instance, even in isolated organs, the administration of the secretion of the adrenal glands, produces changes characteristic of the expression of fear. Sherrington[7] has shown how in dogs, who have been subjected to high division of the spinal cord, so that all the viscera are dissociated so far as nervous influence is concerned, the perception of the adequate stimuli induce all the expressions of fear, anger, etc. It would seem, therefore, that an emotion, as this term is commonly understood, is the psychic aspect of an activation induced by certain stimuli which spreads through both central and vegetative neurones, and influences the secretions of the endocrine glands; and that none of the resulting activities precede, or have a causal relationship to, the rest. The real point to note is that the pattern of stimuli may be in the environment, and start off the activation of the complex pattern through the exteroceptors; or it may be within the body, starting off the activation through the enteroceptors. This allows for emotion, and the accompanying behaviour, arising both through alterations in postural tonus, as described by Kempf, and also in response to environmental stimuli. It is clear that the combinations in such a complex pattern, as is involved in central and autonomic neurones and endocrine glands, may be legion, and hence the varieties and shades of emotion may be legion. James very much objects to the long catalogues of emotions drawn out by certain German psychologists, and yet there is a good deal to support their contention, that there are a very large number of distinct emotional entities which can be discriminated one from the other. The doctrine of emergence accounts for this, for each different combination will emerge with a quality of its own, according to the special relatedness enjoyed. It may be, as James suggests, dry-as-dust reading to wade through lists of these; so it would be to go through the list of possible combinations from the distillation of coal tar, and for descriptive purposes it is useful to classify them more roughly into groups, yet this does not alter the fact that these differences do exist. It may be that in the field of emotions it is only the feeling type who can properly discriminate the different shades and varieties of affect, yet descriptions and enumeration of them may not be without use. To sum up, there can be no doubt that Kempf's contribution to the study of Personality is a very important one, though we cannot accept his contention that all behaviour is determined solely by the affective cravings of autonomic segments. However, it is remarkable how in the study of normal persons, their life works out in accordance with their own bent, often in spite of the environment. How often do people say that fate or luck worked out in such a way, that they have been enabled to follow out some line of work, or they may attribute their fortune to a beneficent personal intervention of the Deity. If these persons' lives are dispassionately criticized, in the vast majority of cases it may be seen that it is they themselves, who consciously, or more often unconsciously strive towards the end they eventually attain, and if this striving is not that of the simple autonomic segments, it is that of the emergence from their combination. Many writers have recognized this inherent guidance of the individual's own life. For example, Maeterlinck says, "Let us not look to the Gods for an explanation of these phenomena. Until these Gods shall have clearly explained themselves, there is nothing that they can explain for us. And destiny, which is merely the God of which we know least, has less right than any of the others to intervene and cry to us, as it does from the depths of its inscrutable night: 'It is I who so willed it!' Nor let us invoke the illimitable laws of the universe, the intentions of history, the will of the worlds, the justice of the stars. These powers exist: we submit to them, as we submit to the might of the sun. But they act without knowing us; and within the wide circle of their influence, a liberty remains to us still, that is probably immense. They have better work on hand, than to be for ever bending over us, to lift a blade of grass or drop a leaf in the little paths of our anthill. Since we ourselves are here the parties concerned, it is, I imagine, within ourselves that the key of the mystery shall be found; for it is probable that every creature carries within him the best solution of the problem that he presents. Within us, underlying the conscious existence that our reason and will control, is a profounder existence, one side of which connects with a past beyond the record of history, the other with a future, that thousands of years cannot exhaust. We may safely conceive, that all the Gods lie hidden within it; that those wherewith we have peopled the earth and the planets will emerge one by one, in order to give it a name and a form, that our imagination may understand. And as man's vision grows clearer, as he shows less desire for image and symbol, so will the number of these names, the number of these forms, tend to diminish. He will slowly arrive at the stage, when there shall be one only that he will proclaim or reserve; when it shall be revealed to him that this last form, this last name, is truly no more, than the last image of a power whose throne was always within him. Then will the Gods that had gone forth from us, be found again in ourselves; and it is there that we will question them to-day."

The spectacle of the square peg in the round hole is all too familiar, and in such a case we have the person whose affective cravings are not strong enough, or insufficiently organized, to overcome the force of the environment, and so he struggles vainly and unhappily against his evil fortune. But the man who is the "right man in the right place" is he, whose cravings are all co-ordinated and integrated in such a way that he goes out to seek and find his proper environment, as certainly and directly as the hungry man, under the impulse of a simple and primitive affective craving, goes out to find a meal. The importance of helping each individual to work out his own salvation is being increasingly recognized by educationists, and the schemes for vocational guidance are the direct outcome of the recognition of the principles underlying behaviour, which Kempf has so admirably enunciated. Moreover, it must be remembered, that although it may be convenient to discuss such questions from the psychological aspect, this is a matter of convenience and nothing more, for a complete description can only be given when the bodily changes, as well as their mental correlates, are determined. To this end Kempf has contributed, and it is probable that the future will acclaim his theses, not as antithetic, but as complementary to the various psychological explanations of behaviour which have been put forward.

CHAPTER XIII

THE INSTABLE PERSONALITY

The Neurotic

A GOOD deal has been said in the last four chapters about neurosis, since the work of the psycho-analytic schools is chiefly concerned with this; and, as has been said, it seems justifiable to consider the instable person while dealing with the subject of personality as a whole, because although the fully developed neurotic and delinquent may justly be regarded as pathological, nevertheless in many respects, a study of such persons' behaviour illustrates tendencies and reactions present in the normal, albeit exhibited in a more crude and exaggerated form. The study of a group of these instable personalities is like studying a series of cartoons. They may be distorted and inartistic, but they do represent many salient features which the orthodox portrait leave unnoticed. There has been a tendency amongst psychologists in the past to paint a picture of the ideal norm, to which none of us attain, and from which the majority of mankind is very far removed. The organization of personality as it should proceed, and would, if it could, has been sketched out in the preceding chapters, and a survey of the failures, and the way they fail, may be instructive, and may explain why all our acquaintances do not emerge on the level of Deity in Alexander's sense. It may be asked, why not proceed a little further, and discuss the insane, who may also illustrate points in the personality of the normal? This argument is apposite to a certain extent, yet there is a marked difference between the normal and the instable on the one hand, and the insane on the other. Apart from structural defects and disease of the brain, the insane person is characterized by the fact that he is not making the least attempt to adapt himself to life, or to aspire to Deity; he accepts the state he is in with pleasure or grief,

P

as the case may be, but makes no effort to change it, nor does he believe that any real change is in any way possible. This is not the natural reaction of the normal personality, nor of the neurotic, both of whom are always striving to find some sort of compromise with their environment which may raise them higher, though the result may not be very satisfactory. The normal person may more or less succeed, and, in so far as he is normal, he is progressive and willing to modify himself as his environment changes. The general law and rhythm, according to which his life proceeds, corresponds to the law and rhythm of universal progress. The behaviour of the insane definitely runs counter to this law and rhythm. The neurotic strives to find this working compromise and fails, either because he is not progressive and tries to fit an old reaction on to a new demand, or because he strives to find a compromise on wrong lines. It is often thought that a neurotic is not trying, and is making no effort. As a rule, this judgment is quite unjust; he is trying very hard, but with so little understanding, and in such wrong directions, that his achievements are almost negligible. The neurotic frequently blames his environment for his lack of success, but in this he deceives himself, for the confusion and conflict which stand in his way lie within himself. His immediate difficulty may be in respect of some incident in his environment, but it is because he is not sufficiently in tune with himself that he cannot adjust himself to it. This may not be directly obvious, even to the onlooker, and still less frequently to the patient himself, yet in practically every case there is too great a discrepancy between what the patient can do, and what he had set before himself as the minimum that he ought to do, and between what he is, and what he would like to be. The patient may try to cover up this discrepancy by persuading himself that he is all that he would like to think. This leads to a self-satisfaction and assertion, which is decidedly objectionable to others, and is not wholly satisfactory to himself, since a doubt of the reality of his estimate is always liable to creep in. Such are the people who are always declaring that their conscience is clear, that they are pure in thought, and not like others, who have nasty minds. In fact it may be that we ought not to dislike that Pharisee, who prayed in the temple and thanked God he was not as other men, but rather to pity him, as at least a potential neurotic, who was striving to cover his knowledge of his own inferiority by a will to power. Still, there probably are people who have succeeded in completely deceiving themselves, and into whose minds doubt never does creep in; on those we need waste no pity. They are within their limits, well organized and adapted to life, at any rate as it appears to them.

Some of the means whereby the neurotic strives to hide from himself his inferiority are of considerable interest, and are recognizable in the behaviour of every one at times. There is a great tendency to project his own qualities on to others so as to detract his own critical attention from himself. To illustrate this projection, an example may be useful. A confidential clerk was once tempted to take some money which did not belong to him. Although he did not actually succumb to the temptation, the recognition of such a possibility in himself was so much at variance with the ideal he had set before himself that it caused him the most acute distress; but he adjusted himself to the situation in the following way. Whereas, before, he had been considerate to his subordinates, and trusted them to do their work in their own way, he became exacting and so suspicious of the honesty and accuracy of the junior clerks that life in the office became perfectly impossible. This tendency to project one's own faults and shortcomings on to others is very common in everyday life, and if we are to be honest with ourselves, we must be very chary when we find that we are judging others, lest we be projecting ourselves in this way. For example, the unprepossessing old maid may honestly think she is striving for the cause of morality when she condemns the flighty ways of her more attractive sisters, but the world at large is apt to suspect the intervention of a slight degree of jealousy. It will be noticed that projection concerns the bad qualities and shortcomings which the neurotic recognizes as positive factors in his make-up. Complementary to this is the phenomenon known as identification, which involves the factors which he recognizes as negative or missing from his make-up. This would seem to involve, as its primary end, the unconscious effort of the neurotic to persuade himself that he is the equal of someone whom he really regards as his superior. The phenomenon manifests itself in all sorts of habits of action, postures, eccentricities of speech and dress, and so on, in which he becomes identical with his ideal. These unconscious minor actions serve as symbols of the major qualities he desires for himself. In ordinary life, this may be exemplified in all sorts of ways, but a good example may be quoted in the following of fashions. If a royalty or person prominent for looks, birth, or other distinction, adopts some style of dress, there is a tendency for others —themselves not leaders of fashion—to identify themselves, by a more or less slavish imitation. Though this process of identification is undoubtedly based on the tendency to imitate, which is inherent in all of us and which has been dealt with above, it represents an emergence at a higher level of organization, in which there is more appreciation of the character as a whole of the person imitated, and an impulse to get into closer personal touch with the latter. The phenomena of true identification unquestionably involve a consciousness of self which is certainly not necessarily involved in imitation. Reactions of identification may be met with, apart from any marked feeling of inferiority in respect of the person with whom identification is achieved. For example, if two friends are discussing a difficult psychological problem, which they are both trying to grasp more clearly, they often find they have adopted identical postures in their chairs, frequently the reverse of comfortable. It is difficult to say which is the imitator and which the imitated, and neither of them is aware of any feeling of inferiority towards the other. These identical postures would seem to be induced rather from an effort to get into more close mental touch with each other, and to achieve a result by an amalgamation of their thoughts, and not by the subjugation of one to another. At the same time, it must be admitted that they both feel a sense of inadequacy, in as much as they are unable to solve the problem by their unaided effort. This phenomenon of identification is closely allied to, and may be well part of that of transference; but this latter term has a definite connotation in relation to the therapeutic process of psycho-analysis, and describes the relationship of patient to physician, so that its discussion here is somewhat out of place, since our aim is to illustrate the personalities of average individuals, rather than to discuss the neurotic for his own sake.

Another refuge is what may be called the plea of "if only." The neurotic may hide behind an illness, real or imaginary, though the word imaginary is probably not really justified. The pains of unpleasant sensations of the neurotic do have a basis in organic changes, which in the normal person would pass unnoticed, or be accepted philosophically as the minor ills to which the flesh is heir. To the sensitive neurotic however, they are felt as major distresses, and their importance is not diminished if these symptoms serve the purpose of excusing them in their own eyes from a task they dare not face. But having established their illness, they are never tired of narrating what they would do if only they were not ill. As a somewhat extreme example of this reaction, we may quote the case of a neurotic girl who had not the courage to enter into the married state, though she was fond enough of her fiancé, and was not averse to the idea of marriage so long as it remained in the distance. One day, however, when trying on her wedding-dress, she fell off her chair, and hurt her leg. She magnified this into a full-dress hysterical illness, and for over forty years never stirred more than a few steps from her bed. But she never ceased from relating to those who would listen, how happy she would have been, and what a wonderful life she would have led, if only she had not been ill. But perhaps she had a cross to bear, for she was forced to live with a younger sister, who wore a monocle, and divided her interest between bridge and horse-racing. From her the patient got scant sympathy. Again the "if only" plea is used in respect of social or financial position, and is the origin of much envious feeling. In this way, the neurotic continually tries to banish from his mind the knowledge that his illness and distress depend on faults within himself. If only he had been born rich, if only his mother had not been delicate, if only he had been brought up in a true religious belief, none of these ills would have come upon him. For all that, from time to time he has uncomfortable flashes of insight in which he sees himself as he really is. To the observer such flashes of insight appear as attacks of deep, and sometimes unreasonable depression. This reaction of flight from self-revelation is one from which few so-called normal people are exempt.

In his struggles to adapt his achievement to his ideal, the neurotic almost inevitably gets discouraged, and with this discouragement his achievements fall below the standard of his real capacity, so that in successful treatment, not only must the ideal be brought down till it is more in accordance with possibilities, but his achievements must be raised, partly by the gain of greater power and capacity, and partly by the removal of the restricting influence of depression.

In general, however, not only are the achievements lowered by depression, but the whole personality sinks back to a lower plane by the process of regression. This regression is not uncommon as a temporary phenomenon in everyday life. The husband or the wife who is not getting his or her way, becomes the spoilt child, is petulant and querulous, or drops back to baby language and even baby tricks. So with the neurotic, for much of his behaviour is that of the spoilt egotistic child. An extreme case of such regression was an ex-sergeant, who came to hospital, unable to articulate a single word, quite ignorant of his identity, his place of abode, his parentage, or whether he was married or not. He could make sounds, so that at first he was thought to be an extreme case of aphasia. But then it was found that in his dreams he could talk quite well; indeed, he used to shout out military orders in such a stentorian voice that some of the other patients, believing themselves back at the front, indulged in the emotional outburst which we describe as a hysterical fit. It was then recognized that he was a case of extreme regression, and that this was due to an overwhelming feeling of inadequacy and failure to meet the situation. As he recovered, he began to talk, much as a baby talks, to cry, when he was disappointed about anything, and to react in a way which was suitable for an infant. However, with the return of his memory he gradually grew up again until he became almost a man. An even more interesting feature of regression is the return along the line of racial, rather than individual history. In this case the behaviour of the patient resembles that of primitive man. His loves and hates and panic fears are not the organized, finely graded emotions of the civilized man, but rather the ill-co-ordinated outbursts of the savage. In his intellectual life, he tends to express himself in symbols, he indulges in elaborate rituals, and transfers his emotional reactions from the big things of life to the lesser things. A good example of this latter tendency is afforded by a spinster lady of early middle life, who constantly got herself entangled with male acquaintances so that she compromised herself and her family, not a little. She refused however to regard herself in any way in the wrong, but made herself almost seriously ill by constantly worrying over trivial things, such as whether she had paid back sixpence lent her by her landlady, or whether she returned a book to a library, or kept it on her own shelves. She transferred her fear of the larger consequences to the small matters, for which she could be visited by no real retribution, just as the primitive transferred his fear of his ancestors and his Gods to his Totem animal, which he could, and sometimes did, kill easily.

The rituals of the primitive who goes through the most complicated rites to appease the hostile Gods, and ward off from himself the consequences of his evil deeds, have their analogue in the washing and other rituals of the neurotic. A woman felt she must wash her hands if ever they touched her body, or even her clothes, which in their turn had come in contact with her body, or she would contaminate any person or thing she touched. Her body was unclean because of a vaginal discharge. This was innocent enough, and had been acquired in an innocent way, but it was associated in her mind with certain incidents in youth which were less in accordance with her moral ideals, and her ritual aimed at purification for the moral sin and the appeasement of the angry Gods. So with Lady Macbeth, "Look how she rubs her hands." "It is an accustomed action with her, to be seen thus washing her hands; I have known her continue in this for a quarter of an hour." Such regressions to rituals and superstitious practices are not uncommon in everyday life when things get too difficult. To illustrate this tendency, we have only to consider the commercial success of quack remedies, and the persuasive powers of such advertisements as that of the rising sun, of a new era of health, and so on. Symbolism is the secret of advertising, and a suggestion of magic, whereby man may attain to the old Eden where he lived in ease and luxury and not by the sweat of his brow, is certain of success.

Many of the physical hysterical symptoms are found to be symbolic in nature, but this is by no means always the case, and an effort to attribute symbolic interpretations to all these symptoms will sometimes lead the investigator very far from the truth. In perhaps the great majority of war cases, for example, these symptoms were the result of suggestion, and were readily curable by counter-suggestion, but they tended to be fixed by the fact that they afforded a means of solution of the problem of how to avoid further service without loss of self-respect. The same is true of many cases in civil life, though in some it is found that there is a symbolic meaning attached to the symptom, which must be resolved before the latter can be removed.

Often this symbolism has relation to a previous experience, of a character analogous to the present difficulty. For example, a lady had set before herself a programme of social work which was quite beyond her capacity, and after a time she was rather suddenly smitten with extreme physical prostration. Rather naturally she was regarded as overworked, and put to bed to rest. Instead of improving, her weakness got so pronounced that she could not sit up in bed. Suggestive methods were tried next, with little or no effect. It was then found that she was experiencing vivid memory pictures of previous experiences with her drunken husband, who had ill-treated her, and whom it had been her chief ambition to reform. Only with difficulty, however, did she remember that on a few occasions she had been prostrated for the whole day after a scene, so that she felt that she could not possibly go on. But once the memory was revived, she could be got to realize the analogy to her present condition, and the symbolic nature of her weakness. She had identified the difficulty of her social work, which could be modified, with the difficulty of reforming her husband, which could not be modified, and had come to regard the achievement of the former as hopeless as the latter. With this realization of this mistaken identification, however, she became quite willing to reduce the demands of her ideal, and from that moment she sat up in bed and steadily regained her strength.

These physical maladies often constitute a compromise which brings momentary satisfaction to the neurotic, so that for the time being the patient seems well content with his condition, but such satisfaction never lasts for long, for the inconvenience of the disability soon gives rise to a desire to be quit of it. Then a new conflict starts, between this desire to recover from the obvious symptom, and the half-conscious fear lest, if he lose his hold on the compromise which has been established, worse may befall him, and he therefore seems to be quite unprepared to give up his disability. These reactions naturally give rise to misunderstandings, and the patient is often looked upon as a malingerer and fraud. This is not the case, and it is only by understanding the true inwardness of the problem that assistance can be rendered and the patient cured. Although these crude regressive symptoms and unsatisfactory compromises may not be met with in the normal person, yet many apparently irrational fears and unexplained impulses are of this nature. Then, too, who is not prone to aches and pains and petty illnesses not to be explained on physical grounds, which may in a small way be used to mitigate the force of circumstances, or excuse the full performance of a duty which seems too hard?

Certain factors in relation to the neuroses require to be considered in somewhat more detail. The first of these is the influence of amnesia, or forgetfulness. McDougall[1] maintains that there can be no neuroses without some degree of amnesia. This is certainly true, but it does not of course explain the whole mechanism of the production of neuroses. For example, it may be true to say that the man with hysterical paralysis of his legs has forgotten how to use them; but this is not the whole story, and the process of recollection may be far from easy. The process of forgetting may be a perfectly conscious act, and for this type Rivers[2] would reserve the term repression, and use suppression to express amnesia which may be induced without the patient being aware of the process. This question of forgetting is dealt with in greater detail in Chapter IX, and need not be referred to again here. Suffice to say, if there is a portion of the personality which has been forgotten, it is not properly associated with the rest, and this dissociation is of the utmost importance in the production of neurotic symptoms and abnormal behaviour. It is probable that amnesic "patches" in the individual make-up are of greater frequency and importance than is generally recognized in normal psychology.

From the point of view of the normal personality, a second factor, namely suggestion and suggestibility is of the utmost importance. The particular nature of the neurotic symptom is determined by suggestion, and many patterns of behaviour in the normal, though they are not neurotic symptoms, are determined in the same way. The acceptance of a suggestion depends on suggestibility. What then do we mean by suggestibility? McDougall defines suggestion as "a process of communication, resulting in the acceptance with conviction of the communicated proposition, in the absence of logically adequate grounds for its acceptance." Following this, we might define suggestibility as a readiness to accept propositions, with a conviction which is not justified by logic and reason.

Formerly, suggestibility was regarded as an abnormal manifestation, but McDougall and others have properly shown that every individual is possessed of this, to a greater or less extent. It is, in fact, an innate tendency of mankind, every individual being born with a capacity to accept suggestion. Like all other innate tendencies, it is greatly modified during the mental growth of the individual, and in the process of the formation of character. Drever[3] has pointed out that suggestibility is very closely bound up with the innate tendency of self-abasement; if indeed, it is not a special manifestation of it. It is quite obvious that the man with a marked degree of the opposite tendency, that of self-assertion, will not readily be suggestible, and later we shall see how this operates in the incidence of suggestibility. We have, then, in each child, a certain tendency to suggestibility, which is modified by the relative preponderance of the disposition of self-abasement and self-assertion. Compared with adults, children are markedly suggestible, but this suggestibility of the child, which is a factor of great utility in his education, is gradually modified till the normal adult reaches his condition of low suggestibility. The young child is extremely dependent on others for all his physical requirements, more particularly, for nutrition and protection from violence. In order that he may gain this advantage, the instinct of self-assertion must be in abeyance, and that of self-abasement in the ascendancy, but as his physical powers increase the child finds that he can do things himself, and that he need no longer depend on others so much, and his self-reliance is developed. Such self-reliance is a complex sentiment, but its basal factor is the disposition of self-assertion, and so with its growth, suggestibility decreases. Again, as suggestibility consists in readiness to accept propositions with a conviction, which is not justified by logic or reason, it follows that the stronger the reasoning powers, and the more readily they can be brought to bear on a new situation, the less will be the suggestibility of an individual. But in order to reason about a subject we must have knowledge about it, and the knowledge must be well organized and well arranged in our minds, if we are to apply it to the new situation. In other words, function must be integrated at a high cortical level, as was seen in Chapter VII. This function only comes into evidence as the child grows into the man.

It is next necessary to consider certain factors which modify a man's suggestibility. Firstly, the subjective factors inherent in man and constituting an individual disposition favourable to suggestion, are youth, inexperience, lack of knowledge of the topic in connexion with which the suggestion is given, and general lack of organized knowledge and settled convictions. Secondly, the subjective factors, originating from external causes, are the low vitality induced by fatigue and sickness, the disturbance produced by the action of the emotions, and the influence of the herd in framing the individual convictions. Thirdly, the objective factors are conditions depending on the source from which the suggestion is given, conditions depending on the manner in which it is given, and conditions depending on the circumstances under which it is given. The second and third groups require further consideration.

The low vitality produced by fatigue and illness is a potent factor in increasing the power of suggestion, and falls within the experience of every one. The reason of this is, that when our vitality is low we feel physically feeble and incapable of acting for ourselves, and so our self-reliance is diminished, and our self-abasement gains ascendancy over our self-assertion. In addition, when fatigued we find we have not our usual power of marshalling the elements of our knowledge. We do not actually lose anything out of our store of known facts, but we cannot recall the requisite data quickly, and so our power of reasoning, and of making quick decisions, is lessened. This interferes with our power of criticizing outside suggestions which are likely to be followed as the line of least resistance. This depends on the diminution in efficient cortical function under the influence of fatigue, which is described below.

In states of extreme emotional disturbances suggestibility is increased, and the more intense the emotional feeling, the greater is the suggestibility. As Drever has pointed out, the intensity of emotional feeling increases with the resistance to the realization of the normal activity, which the individual should exhibit, as a result of the emotion. Hence a man who is in a situation in which a powerful emotion, such as fear or anger, is aroused, but where the normal activities of flight or attack are prevented, tends to be very highly suggestible. The reason for this is that an intense emotion dominates the whole consciousness, crowding out principles, reason, logic, and all higher thought activities, so that a suggestion coming from the outside finds no resistance to its activities and has a clear field to work upon. As has been seen, this crude emotional activity depends on activation at thalamic levels, the normal cortical control and inhibition being in abeyance. In addition, there is considerable endocrine disturbance, which may inhibit cortical function. If a suggestion can be brought to bear on the subconscious fields of the mind without due intervention of full consciousness, it will be much more potent, because no reason is brought to bear upon it. This is most obvious in the potency of suggestions given to a patient under hypnosis, when the appeal is entirely to processes on the subconscious level. It is also seen in the condition just referred to, for the emotion occupies the whole field of consciousness.

The influence of the herd has a great power of increasing the suggestibility of the individual. Man is a gregarious animal, and in all his ideas and actions is influenced by the dictates of the herd. People hold convictions and regulate their behaviour to a great extent because their " set " think and act like that, and to think or act differently is " not the thing." Even in the case of social rebels, who would appear to be exceptions to this rule, they are found to be members of a small clique within the greater herd, and adhere even more closely to the dictates of this small coterie than do the members of the larger herd to their code of social ethics. There can be no doubt that the very fact of being suggestible to the dictates of a community renders the individual less suggestible to influences coming from outside the herd, but this does not alter the fact that the more closely an individual is bound up in a community, the more suggestible he becomes. The factor underlying this suggestibility is the feeling of self-abasement of the individual in face of the composite force of the whole community, and the fact that he is frequently forced to accept situations in which his individual reasoning powers are not allowed to act. In other words, his cortical function of discrimination is not allowed full development, and so, subcortical function is permitted to influence his action. This suggestibility is well seen in the behaviour of crowds, more particularly when it is increased by the presence of intense emotion. Hence an orator is able to sway a crowd to his will, if he first arouses the emotions of its members, and then instils suggestion. It is to be noted, however, that he must be, or pretend to be in sympathy with the general opinion of the crowd to begin with, so that he appears to be speaking from within the herd, otherwise he will tend to arouse opposition rather than compliance.

It would seem that hysterical symptoms, as well as much of the suggested behaviour of normal persons, may be produced as a result of six sets of circumstances, and in each of these it is necessary to define the psychical influence which increases the suggestibility, and the physical influence which determines the nature of the symptom or behaviour. Probably in all cases, both factors operate to a certain extent, but their relative preponderance varies enormously, for in some cases the psychical factor, by markedly increasing the suggestibility of the patient, allows a relatively slight physical suggestion to be perpetuated as a hysterical symptom, or to materially alter the individual's behaviour in life; while in other cases, the physical suggestion is so strong that the symptom will be impressed on a person of relatively low suggestibility. It is convenient to arrange the groups of hysterical symptoms in such an order as will represent descending grades of psychical suggestibility.

The first group is found in those people, who have acquired a sense of inferiority, either in respect of their whole body, or of one or more limbs or organs. In such persons, who are almost hypochondriacal in their expectation of illness, the slightest physical accident, or passing ache or pain, is sufficient to determine a hysterical symptom, either affecting the whole body, or a particular limb or organ, which is believed to be weak. The treatment has not been completed when the hysterical symptom has been removed, or the particular reaction of behaviour altered, for the suggestibility is in this case pathological, and the mental derangement, which has determined this, must be put right. Here the suggestibility depends on the abnormal preponderance of the tendency to self-abasement which makes these patients consider themselves inferior to others. The mental processes of such people are extremely complex, for the two reactions of self-abasement and self-assertion are by no means mutually exclusive, and we may find the patient displaying extreme self-abasement in one direction, but considerable self-assertion in another as is discussed above, in dealing with the will to power. Another factor which increases the suggestibility in these persons is that their lack of mental integration prevents them using their reasoning and critical powers to full advantage, and so they are unable to examine the value of the physical cause of their hysterical symptoms. Further, as their condition progresses they get really ill, and their vitality is lowered so that they become more suggestible, while the emotion of self-pity, which is aroused, works still further in the same direction. In such cases the hysterical symptom may be of any variety, as the slightest physical stimulus will be responded to.

In the next group, the hysterical symptoms are sequelæ of commotion. Here some actual physical trauma, such as a blow on the head, has, without necessarily causing complete loss of consciousness, led to general confusion of the patient's mind. This may lead to a very temporary inability to hear, or see, or remember. Under such circumstances the patient's suggestibility is increased by the complete abolition of the power of reasoning and criticizing. The full conscious state is temporarily unattainable, and impressions are made only on his subconscious mind, which is always more amenable to suggestion. Under such circumstances, the fact that he cannot hear, see, or remember, suggests to him that he must be deaf, blind or have lost his memory. Having received this suggestion, he ceases to listen, to look, or to try to remember, so that until he is treated, he is hysterically deaf, blind or amnesic. These three hysterical symptoms have been quoted because they are the most characteristic of this group, but paralysis, dumbness, and other hysterical manifestations, may result under the same circumstances. These two groups apply more particularly to pathological states, but they may serve to complete the illustration of the way in which suggestions act on the normal individual.

In the third group, the symptoms are produced under

stress of great emotion. In such cases, as the natural outlet of the emotion is blocked, the intensity of the emotional feeling increases with the flow of activity through vegetative neurones. With this, the physical expressions of emotion, which are useful in their incipient stages, become useless if they are intensified by the concentration of activation in visceral patterns, so that the muscular activity, which ought to be used in the performance of the normal active sequel of the emotion, is wasted in secondary expressions of emotion. On the pathological side, such symptoms are dumbness and stammering, rigidity, tremor, and collapse of the legs, and excessive purposeless movements; these physical phenomena are perpetuated as hysterical mutism, stammering, tremor and paraplegia, and in the case of the purposeless movements, as hysterical tics or fits. The increased suggestibility is determined by the complete domination of the emotion, and the consequent loss of reasoning powers and cortical function generally. In the case of fear, under the stress of which hysterical symptoms are specially prone to develop, there is definite self-abasement in the presence of some overwhelming situation. In the case of panics or mob anger, the suggestibility may also be increased by the influence of the herd, as was discussed above, but this would be in a general rather than in a particular way.

In the next group, the symptoms are produced by hetero-suggestion. Such may be illustrated as follows: In hysterical cases, fresh disabilities are sometimes produced as the result of some unwise remark or action on the part of the physician or nurse, which conveys to the patient the suggestion that he has some physical disability. Several psychical factors come into play. Firstly, there is the relative self-abasement which the patient feels in the presence of the physician, especially in respect of his knowledge of the subject. Secondly, his own lack of organized knowledge will itself prevent proper criticism of the suggestion. Then, we have objective factors, such as the prestige of the physician, the manner in which he makes the remark, and the circumstances under which it is made. For example, if a distinguished doctor remarks in the presence of an assembly of other physicians, all apparently agreeing, that the patient may have a disease which will result in paralysis of both legs, the suggestion may be accepted, and paraplegia will develop. Or again, if a physician, very carefully and with considerable ceremony, examines for anæsthesia, asking if the patient feels this and that, the patient thinks he is expected to have anæsthesia, and will readily develop it. How this hetero-suggestion acts in altering the behaviour of the normal individual is too familiar to require discussion. We have only to consider the power of the press, and the stump orator, and how the reaction is made use of in ordinary education to realize its importance.

In the fifth group, we have to deal with behaviour acquired by imitation from another person. The physical stimulus is here more defined, and symptoms such as stammering, abnormal movement, and various gaits, seen in other patients are acquired. The psychical stimulus in this case is due to self-abasement felt by the imitator in face of another person whom he regards as very wonderful or very extraordinary, and a certain interference with the critical powers, induced by the emotion of curiosity and the influence of the herd. Here, however, the psychical element is of much less importance, for the tendency to imitate is strong in us all, and it does not require much extra suggestibility to determine the perpetuation of the imitative symptom, which quickly becomes a habit. The acquisition of accents, tricks of speech and behaviour is very familiar in normal persons, and has already been discussed in relation to identification.

In the last group are comprised symptoms which are habit continuations of definite, but temporary organic disabilities, and as such, are more or less confined to pathological cases. Such symptoms may range from blindness and deafness, through vomiting and urinary troubles, to paralysis, contractures and anæsthesias. Here the physical stimulus is enormously strong, for it is actually present in the patient's own body. The psychical factor of increased suggestibility is present to a slight degree, and may be induced by low vitality, owing to the illness, and to a failure of a unification of all the wishes of the personality towards recovery. This applies not only to these major disabilities, but also to the minor aches and pains which are of such everyday occurrence as to be almost included within the limits of normal experience.

To sum up, suggestibility is a factor of enormous importance in determining the nature and reactions of the personality. It essentially depends on a temporary or permanent failure of integration, and of what we have come to regard as high level cortical activity. Furthermore, under the influence of suggestion, the individual will tend to react more and more at low levels and will exercise his functions of discrimination and control to a less and less extent.

It will be clear from the above, that acceptance of suggestions, not only is induced by, but also leads to a condition of dissociation in the patient's mind. This state of dissociation is regarded by Janet[4] as the essential factor in the neurosis, and this coincides with the initial contention of this chapter, that it was a dissociation in the personality, between the ideal and the reality. This state of dissociation is fully discussed in Chapter XV. In any case, the failure of proper association and organization of the personality marks a failure of function of the highest levels of the cortex. This is perpetuated by the establishment of a vicious circle, through the influence of fatigue, and reference to this may serve to illustrate once more our contention that the neuroses and psychoses, in Huxley's sense, are different aspects of the same essential process.

There can be no question that many of the symptoms of neurotics, and some of the atypical behaviour of normal people, are the direct result of fatigue. Such fatigue may be produced by physical overwork, though this is rare, or by mental overwork on the conscious or at the unconscious level. Fatigue, however, as has been shown, is not an explanation of the neurotic state in itself. This is why the old-fashioned rest cure, in cases of neuroses, is frequently inadequate. So long as the fatigue is due to friction between the personality as a whole and the outside world, then the removal of the friction by isolation of the ego allows for the necessary recuperation, and recovery results. When, on the other hand, the fatigue is the result of friction within the ego, then mere rest is not enough, for the friction still persists, and cure does not ensue. It is a truism in neurology, that the higher structures are more readily fatigued than those of lower levels; naturally therefore the functions of the highest level structures suffer first and most severely, from any process of fatigue. As we have seen in Chapter IV, the highest grade of structure in man is the cerebral cortex, and the functions of this aggregation of cells are upset by the processes of fatigue, earlier and more markedly than are the other functions of the body.

The conceptions of these functions have changed not a little in recent years. With the tremendous impetus given to anatomical and histological study, by the improvements in optical and electrical methods which took place in the last half of the nineteenth century, it seemed possible that the researches of such workers as Ferrier and Wernicke would lead to a mapping out of the whole cortex into geographical areas, each of which would be found to correspond to a definite function connected with definite parts of the body. More recent work, however, has turned attention in other directions. Exact anatomical correspondence can no longer be regarded as part of the business of the cortex, though it is of course quite clear that certain areas have to do with certain major functions of the body, such as motion, sensation and the work of the distance receptors involving vision and hearing and so on. In these relations the functions to which cortical structure is essential are control, integration, discrimination and reference in time and space, as we have seen.

It is remarkable that the behaviour of neurotics is mainly characterized by deficiency in what we have learnt to regard as the chief functions of the cortex. To take a few examples. In hysterical paralysis, it is movements that are impeded, not individual muscular action. It is characteristic of hysterical pain that the reaction, in some ways, resembles that seen in the thalamic syndrome, in which cortical control is absent. The behaviour of neurotics always tends to be of the "all or none" variety. This is especially true of their emotional reactions, which closely resemble those of Bianchi's monkeys.[5] Their undiscriminated anxieties and fears are primitive affective reactions, in no way co-ordinated into properly organized emotions and sentiments, and the resolution of these by the processes of psycho-therapy essentially involves their proper discrimination and correlation. In the case of the obsessions, the salient feature is the want of accurate reference in time and space. So much is this so, that it is only by restoring the proper time-space relationship of these symptoms that they can be removed.

This may serve to indicate that the immediate precursor of neurotic symptoms is the abrogation of cortical function, and that this failure of function is to a certain extent due to the action of fatigue products. This conception does not run counter to other explanations of neurotic symptoms such as dissociation, for the most marked forms of dissociation of function are those produced when the associative function of the cortex is in abeyance. Indeed, it is clear that a properly associated personality is only possible when the cortex is intact. It is, of course, the duty of the physician not to be content with this explanation of symptom, but to strive to discover the true cause of the fatigue; by this means only will he cure the disease and not merely remove the symptom. None the less the recognition that fatigue of the cortex is an important factor in this connexion is salutary, since it will tend to broaden the outlook of the physician, and prevent his applying only one method of treatment to all cases of neuroses. He will remember that fatigue may be induced by mental conflict, by a prolonged toxæmia, by endocrine disturbance, and by overwork, and so he is less likely to miss his view of the wood by too great concentration on individual trees.

So with the normal personality, fatigue may often be the direct precursor of variation from what is regarded as normal behaviour, but this fatigue is not always produced simply from overwork, and the student must look further than this to understand why certain people show signs of fatigue more readily than others. It is probably true that hard work alone seldom did anyone much harm, in absence of worry and conflict. In any case, the point to be noted is that interference with the proper function of cortical cells by the poisons of fatigue does produce all sorts of mental abnormalities of the most complicated character.

While discussing the neurotic, certain remarks on the "artistic temperament," or more accurately, the "artistic personality" are not out of place. Artists are not generally regarded as pathological, but are essentially instable in Trotter's sense, and only too frequently neurotic. There is the same want of stability, the same want of full conscious control, the same abnormal integrations, which are activated, and which form new emergents, as the thoughts and actions of genius. These new emergents are not predictable, and may show the most banal futilities, or the most transcendently original conceptions.

Indeed, many of the finest achievements of thought have their origin below the level of consciousness. That is to say that they are not integrated and built up in accordance with reason and logic and full cortical function.

William James[7] has shown this in the case of religious experience, Jung in the case of a great generalization in physics—namely Mayer's theory of the Conservation of Energy—and according to Nietzsche and Schopenhauer, this is the case even with philosophy. "Academic" psychologists, such as Souriau and Paulham, admit this by implication, while the psycho-analytic studies of Maeder[8] and Pfister[9] have assigned to unconscious processes a great influence in artistic creation. In addition we find more idealistic thinkers, like Dr Geley,[10] who boldly says of artist or savant that he "ne dirige pas l'inspiration ; il la subit."

Pfister cites the example of a savant achieving his results by inspiration, in the person of Kékulé, who discovered the benzol ring in chemical combinations. While working at the elucidation of the benzol theory, Kékulé found himself in difficulties, and describes how one day he fell into a dreamy state on the top of an omnibus when, suddenly, the solution appeared before him in a sort of picture in which snake-like movements played a large part, which was in reality a regression towards an infantile form of thinking, strictly comparable to the pseudo-hallucination of neurotics.

Nor do mathematical discoveries form an exception, as Dwelshauvers[11] shows by quoting Henri Poincaré, the French mathematician. The latter attributed the solution of many of his particular problems to unconscious action and to "sensibilité" rather than to reason. *Apropros* of this "étât affectif," Dwelshauvers adds, "La démonstration qui s'élabore inconsciémment, est celle, qui a la plus d'affinité avec notre sentiment esthétique. C'est donc la vie des sentiments, qui est ici déterminante. Seules les combinaisons, qui nous émeuvent s'imposent a la conscience et fixent l'attention. Or, il arrive que ce, qui plaît au sens esthétique, apporte en même temps un aide efficace a l'esprit. La solution la plus belle est aussi la plus harmonieuse, et son harmonie est d'un grand secours pour la pensée. L'inconscient est donc ici le processus d'affinité entre notre sensibilité et l'invention." This feeling of appropriateness is a common feature with mathematicians. "Les combinaisons utiles, ces sont precisément les plus belles, je veux dire celles qui peuvent le mieux charmer cette sensibilité speciale, que tous les mathematiciens connaissent" writes Poincaré.

So it is not surprising, that poets and painters also should have felt intuitively the source of their ideas to be outside consciousness, and to have felt inspiration surge up mysteriously.

For example, Goethe, in writing to von Humboldt, speaks of great thought in one's power, but due to a superior force to which a man yields unconsciously; also elsewhere " Alles ist als wie geschenkt." Schiller (quoted by Pfister) says: " the unconscious with discretion makes the poetic artist." De Musset writes: " On ne travaille pas, on écoute, on attende. C'est comme un inconnu qui vous parle a l'oreille." In similar strain Charlotte Brontë in the preface to her sister Emily's *Wuthering Heights*, says, " But this I know; the writer who possesses the creative gift, owns something of which he is not always master — something that, at times, strangely wills and works itself. . . .

". . . As for you—the nominal artist—your share in it has been to work passively under dictates, you neither delivered, nor could question—that would not be uttered at your prayer, nor suppressed nor changed at your caprice. If the result be attractive, the world will praise you, who little deserves praise; if it be repulsive, the same world will blame you, who almost as little deserve blame."

Amongst painters, we find intuitive use of subconscious activities when Leonardo bids his pupils obtain suggestions from stains on walls, which, like Blake's gazing into the fire, is a method of allowing the ever active unconscious processes to be perceived by consciousness, and no painter more frankly turns to the stirrings of his unconscious mind for inspiration, than did Blake.

Passing by the methods adopted by artists such as Titian and Corot (and a hundred others)—where they turned pictures to the wall when for the moment there is no more to say, but reverted later to the work, as suggestions from the unconscious mind came to their help in the process of building up the composition—one may quote a modern painter of great influence and personality, namely Gauguin, who vividly describes his experience in painting his great picture " D'où venons nous? Que sommes nous? Où allons nous?" He says " Ou commence l'execution d'un tableau, où finit elle? Au moment où des sentiments extrêmes sont en fusion au plus profond de l'être, au moment où ils éclatent, et que toute la pensee sort comme la lave d'un volcan, n'y a-t-il pas là une éclosion de l'œuvre soudainement creee, brutale si l'on veut, mais grande et d'apparence surhumaine? Les froids calcules de la raison n'ont pas preside a cette éclosion, mais, qui sait, quand au fond de l'être l'œuvre a été commencée? inconsciente peut-étre?" Whistler put this tersely when he said, "Art just happens."

From the foregoing it is clear that many artists have realized that their achievements are not the result of rational laboured thought processes, of which they are aware, but that they sprang from some source, as to whose nature and limitations they had but a hazy idea; and in such processes, we have a close analogy to neurotic symptoms, in the absence of higher cortical functions. How then can we differentiate between the futilities of the psychasthenic and the glorious achievement of a Titian and a Leonardo? Two factors seem to be of importance in this respect. In the first place, if we take the full appearance of cortical function as the highest level in our hierarchy, we may recognize several levels of behaviour before we reach this stage of complete absence of cortical function. This may be explained by the fact that not only is the cortex in man enormously enlarged and complicated, in respect of its area, when compared to that of animals, but also there is the further differentiation to be taken into account of the increase in the layers of cells. There is considerable evidence to show that the more superficial layers subserve the higher functions. Hence, this allows for many degrees of devolution from the highest levels of control, and the process of artistic emergence may well be derived from a level considerably higher than are the emergents which represent neurotic behaviour. In the second place, although artistic expression may arise from subconscious levels, if it is to be of value it must be subjected to considerable modifications by fully conscious function, whereas, in the case of neurotic behaviour, the discipline of this function may not be enjoyed. Indeed, in the genius we may observe a temporary dissociation of cortical function, as if the lower levels could first be freed from its restricting influence, and then the resulting products rigidly subjected to it. For example, this distinction occurs amongst artists, for the greatest geniuses always subject their creations to the most loving care and attention until they are satisfied that their work is perfect in their own eyes. This leads us to the definition of genius as an infinite capacity for taking pains, which, at first sight, seems contradictory to the conception of genius as the flair for seeing things differently from the ordinary mortal. If we consider those artists who work while the inspiration is upon them but immediately after this is over take no more pains or interest in their creation, we find that they may produce original work, but never work of the highest merit. The artist must be essentially subjective, and at least in certain of his attitudes, introvert. If he were completely extravert and objective, then he would merely copy and he would not be a true artist, who must infuse into his work something of himself. It does not follow that he is preponderantly introvert, for many of the greatest artists, such as Goethe and Shakespeare, were unquestionably extraverts, but, as has been said, extraversion and introversion are only attitudes, and though extravert in his attitude to objects, the artist must add something of his own creative effort to the impressions he obtains from the external world. This creative effort may be expressed, from the psycho-physical standpoint, by saying that the engrams which subserve his behaviour are so formed that emergents arise, which are not exactly adapted to the world as it is, but constitute a new and fresh orientation. In this connexion, it should be noticed that we are apt to regard perfect adaptation to the environment as it is, as the highest level of function, thus laying stress on the cortical functions of integration and control and, perhaps, not giving enough attention to discrimination. If this function of complete adaptation were really achieved, progress would be impossible, and that is why the artist and the genius, instable though they may be, are essential to society. Further, if we regard adaptation to the environment as it is, as the summit of achievement, we are presuming that the environment has reached a stabilized perfection. This is obviously untrue, and our own failures in adaptation may be the chief means of progress, inasmuch as they make for a change in the environment. By all the laws of evolution both we and our environment are engaged on the march of progress, and the instability of the genius and the neurotic is due to their being out of step with the environment; the former half a pace in advance, while the latter is half a pace behind. None the less, an accident is always liable to happen whereby they change places, for this progress is not as it were, in one dimension only, but in several. Thus, even the average man may be in step in several dimensions but half a pace behind in one, and half a pace in front in another. It will depend, therefore, on what dimension is significant for the moment, whether he is normal, neurotic, or a genius.

Such a brief exposition naturally cannot cover the whole ground, but may serve to indicate how it is that "genius is akin to madness," and why it is that the artist is so frequently ill-fitted to meet the world. Moreover, it may show that though a personality is instable, he is not necessarily useless, and that many neurotic personalities might have been, and may, under favourable circumstances, still be honoured members of society, instead of being despised, both by the world and by themselves.

CHAPTER XIV

THE INSTABLE PERSONALITY

The Delinquent

IN our study of the instable personality, as exemplified by the neurotic, we have suggested that his inability to cope with life is due to an intrinsic conflict, which may be partly inherent and partly the product of circumstances. In the case of the delinquent, he may or may not be neurotic, but the main stress of conflict is not so much within the ego, as between the ego and the environment. We must ask first, however, what justification there is for supposing that there is a special type of personality who tends to be delinquent? Lombroso[1] and others have insisted that it is possible to recognize a criminal type, even from the physical aspect of anthropology. Goring,[2] on the other hand, in his elaborate empirical study of the English convict, has refuted this claim; he says, "both with regard to measurements and the presence of physical anomalies in criminals, our statistics present a startling conformity with similar statistics of the law-abiding classes. This final conclusion we are bound to accept, until further evidence, in the train of long series of statistics, may compel us to reject or to modify an apparent certainty—indeed our inevitable conclusion must be, that there is no such thing as a physical criminal type." Although there may be no definite stigmata, however, he notes that, "taken as a whole, all English criminals, with the exception of those technically convicted of fraud, are markedly differentiated from the general population, in stature and body weight; while offenders convicted of violence to the person are characterized by a degree of strength, and of constitutional soundness, considerably above the average of other criminals and of the law-abiding community. Thieves and burglars (who constitute, it must be borne in mind, 90 per cent. of all criminals) and also incendiaries, as well as being inferior in stature and weight, are also, relatively to other criminals and the population at large, puny in their general bodily habit. These are the facts; and, according to the results of our statistical enquiry, they are the sole facts, at the basis of criminal anthropology; they are the only elements of truth, out of which have been constructed the elaborate, extravagant and ludicrously uncritical criminological doctrines of the great protagonist of the criminal type theory."

He concludes further, that various physical diseases are not correlated with crime, but that there is a high degree of relationship between criminality and insanity, alcoholism and venereal disease. These three, we may note, are the products of instability. "The one significant physical association with criminality is a general defective physique. The one vital mental constitutional factor, in the etiology of crime, is defective intelligence." The first offence of a criminal is almost always theft, and this, with sex offence, are the crimes characteristic of youth. He notes the importance of the incipient appearances of crime in the young, and remarks, "crime makes its appearance in childhood, just as intellectual capacities, etc., appear at this time; so do many diseases, such as measles, appear in childhood." He lays great stress on inheritance, and on the origin of crime in the constitution of the malefactor, and especially in his mental defective constitution. He states, "criminal diathesis is inherited at much the same rate as are other physical and mental qualities and pathological conditions in man. The influence of parental contagion is inconsiderable, relatively to the influence of inheritance and of mental defectiveness." It must be remembered however, that Goring wrote at a time when heredity was very much in vogue, and when the importance of early environmental influences were little understood. More stress would be laid nowadays on the effect of this early environment in moulding for good or ill the mind of the young child. More recent writers such as Healey[8] are emphatic, that "born criminals" is a misleading term. "Mental defectives and epileptics, and others, especially if brought up in bad environment, may be regarded as having secondary criminal dispositions, but calling them born criminals tells us nothing of worth concerning them." As Devon says, the criminal is just as much, or just as little, born and made, as the policeman is born and made.

These authorities are agreed that there is no one causative factor for delinquency, but rather that we must look for the interaction of several influences. These influences will not be found exclusively in the heredity, nor yet exclusively in the environment; and, if they are to be understood and in any way modified, they must be studied in the child. What leads to criminality would seem to be a difficulty in the adaptation to circumstances, which constitutes the highest function of man's mind, and which gives him so much more control over his medium than is enjoyed by the rest of the animal world. Although the general social environment is of great importance, it is the particular subtle action of the environment on a given individual, that is really influential. Such general influences as bad housing, insanitary surroundings, and so on, may or may not be important, but are only so in respect to the particular individual who may be the subject of our study. We have to solve the question as to why one child, out of several in a community or a family, fails to adapt himself and to grow up a normal law-abiding citizen. The variation must be in the child, since the other factor is nearly constant, and this variation may be inherent, or may be induced by disease, or faulty influences brought to bear on him in his home during the impressionable years before he went to school. In the normal child, the personality is integrated, so that a more or less simple facet is presented to the environment and a minimum of friction results. In the delinquent child, this facet is not smooth, but complex and unequal, and therefore friction is at a maximum. Integration is poor, and therefore adaptation is hindered. As we have said, in the neurotic the instability would seem to lie within the ego, and secondarily between himself and the environment, while in the delinquent, the instability is chiefly, if not primarily, between himself and the environment.

This failure of integration may be due to many causes, and we must attempt to enunciate and exemplify these, in order to throw light on our first problem as to why the delinquent child is delinquent; but even this study will only solve the question incompletely, for it may be possible to quote case for case, in which the so-called causative factors are apparently identical and yet no delinquent behaviour results. Nevertheless this is analogous with the observations noted above in Chapter III, where it was pointed out, that causative factors were not the only determinants of resultant emergents, but that the special relatedness of these factors was of primary importance. The exact nature of this relatedness at the levels of life and consciousness is still beyond our ken, so that we cannot yet wholly determine what makes a criminal and what makes an honest man. Adequate integration depends on perfect cortical function at its highest levels, and such perfect functioning is only possible if there is perfect structural development. When this is not achieved as the result of arrest of development, we are faced with the problem of mental deficiency. The extreme degrees of this condition are not important in relation to delinquency, for such cases are easily recognized, and are, in accordance with legal requirements, put into an environment which is more or less suitable, and which is largely made to fit their needs, since it is recognized that they cannot be expected to adapt themselves to ordinary school or social life. Thus, amongst convicted delinquents, Burt[4] and others have shown that not more than 7 per cent. come within the limits of certifiable feeble-mindedness. However, when we have to deal with children who are merely backward, we find such a condition a fruitful source of delinquency. The backward child is a poorly integrated personality, and he is therefore suggestible, and likely to respond to any influence which is operative at the moment. Moreover, he is not fitted to adapt himself to his environment, however hard he may try. This means that his work at school is done by fits and starts, unless a master of specially strong character achieves an influence over him and induces him to resist other suggestions to take the easier path and avoid work. It may be, however, that the strong influence which rules him, is for evil and not for good, and this may lead him to join a gang who frequently put the dirty work of their nefarious schemes on to their victim. Such children frequently appear in the juvenile courts, accused of crimes to which they have been instigated by their more wicked, but more astute confederates. Unless dominated by a strong personality, however, the backward child will tend to drift, never concentrating long on one thing, achieving little and becoming easily discouraged. If self-assertive, there will be a constant effort to persuade himself that he is as good as his neighbour, and if he cannot achieve success in one way, he will do so in another. However, his frequent failure will lead to a deep sense of inferiority, and the development of a compensatory will to power. Apart from mental defect this sense of inferiority is of enormous importance. It may be induced by a real or fancied mental inferiority, by physical weakness, or a failure to excel in particular games, or by a real or fancied moral defect. Thus, many boys are found to have a sense of inferiority because they fancy that the fact that they have practised masturbation has set them apart from all other boys, has branded them as degenerates, and so on. This sense of inferiority, whatever its origin, saps the whole of a child's ambition and so renders his achievement far less than it might have been, if his performance had reached the limit of his capacity. Everything seems useless, so why try? Again, as has been shown by Adler, various physical inferiorities, whether of the whole body, or of particular organs, lead to similar self-depreciation and, amongst better-class children, the importance attached to games in the public schools leads to an inferiority feeling if there is marked deficiency in this respect, quite apart from general physical prowess. Such deficiency may be due to poor muscular co-ordination and control, to bad sight or hearing, and so, these defects may have a secondary influence in determining an effort to excel somehow or other, and the only way may be by crime. This tendency is often reinforced by the fact that these handicapped children, like all other children, are given to hero-worship, and the formation of ideals. The choice of this ideal may not be overwise, and even if it is commendable, the personality may be so different from his own, that any degree of identification with the ideal is impossible, and the failure to achieve this only leads to more self-depreciation. Naturally, the child often takes his father for his ideal, and in this case, it is hard for him to emulate the adult, for their circumstances and opportunities are so utterly different. This discrepancy between subject and ideal is especially marked if the latter has died when the former was young. For example, a boy made an absolute ideal of his father, and this idealism was intensified since his mother had died in his infancy. To his ten-year-old eyes, this father, a fine type of soldier, of a religious frame of mind, was all that a man could possibly be, strong, brave, holy and honourable. Then the father was killed in the first year of the war.

As the boy grew older and went through school, every time he was not perfectly brave, perfectly honourable, and perfectly strong, he felt he had failed without hope of redemption and, because he could not take a serious interest in religion, he felt he must be an abandoned soul. It mattered not that his companions were as weak as he. The real standard for him was the exaggerated picture of his father, who was as much above him and beyond him at eighteen, as he had been at ten. Under more normal circumstances, as the son gets older, the discrepancy between himself and his father gets less and less, and it may not be an unmixed curse that the godlike parent is discovered to have feet of clay. The sense of inferiority once established, may remain like a millstone round his neck, dragging the child back, so that he fails to expand his personality to meet the more complicated demands of advancing years. Thus, as he becomes less and less adapted to his surroundings, he becomes more and more difficult and, with a chance association with bad environment, he may easily be precipitated into a life of crime. As has been said, if he is of a self-assertive type he may try to compensate for his inferiority by the development of a will to power. By this is meant a striving to excel in some way, whether in reality or phantasy. If success is striven for in reality, and this is denied him in work and games, the child may seek other means of satisfaction. Such means are often sexual, whether by the spreading of undesirable information, or by more active practices. The former is exemplified by a backward girl, who had to be removed from more than one school because she persisted in surrounding herself with an admiring and respectful audience to whom she related sexual details, gleaned from a not less backward elder sister. The latter type may be exemplified by an unpopular boy, who became head of his school-house, but who had to be expelled because he was found sexually abusing other boys, by which means he sought to curry favour, and at the same time achieve for himself a sense of superiority. That this will to power, secondary to a sense of inferiority, is responsible for much bullying, goes without saying. Sometimes, the will to power is achieved in phantasy, rather than in reality. For example, a boy got an order for a shirt, signed by his house-master, but rubbed out the word "shirt," and substituted a whole first eleven kit. These garments he could never wear, but presumably he wished to gloat over them and think of what might have been. Mrs Delafield has given the world an interesting and able study of this sort of case in her book *Reversion to Type.* Sometimes such backward children, who go wrong, are called moral imbeciles, but this term, though it may be convenient, should not be retained in a scientific vocabulary. There is no special faculty of morality which is deficient in these children, but there is either a general backwardness, leading to lack of integration, or some form of imbalance, such as is described below, which will result in the same deficiency. The inefficient child is, therefore, liable to become delinquent, not so much because of his backwardness *per se*, but because he is compelled to live in school, or in work, where it is impossible for him to adapt himself. Take such a child early enough, before the success of his delinquent behaviour has induced too great facilitation of this pattern, and put him in an environment to which he can adapt himself and he does not grow into a criminal.

Passing from the mental deficient, the proper development of cortical function may be interfered with by disease. Epilepsy is important in this respect, for in this condition, apart from the fits, there is an increasing failure of higher mental integration and adaptation, a progressive narrowing of the field of personality, so that the subject becomes more and more egocentric, more and more difficult. Though this characteristic may be more marked as life advances, yet the epileptic child presents such a problem, that quite apart from the disturbance created by his fits, he cannot readily be kept in the ordinary school or workshop. He soon becomes a social rebel, since the demands of self-sacrifice made by society interfere with his characteristic egocentricity. From this it is a short step to the mental state in which the idea of vengeance on society becomes dominant, and from this such crimes as theft and arson often originate, if the impulse does not lead further to crimes of violence against fancied enemies. In such cases, too, we have at times to deal with automatisms, phases during which all conscious control is in abeyance, and the subject may perform acts dictated by his lower level impulses, which may often lead him into a social and even criminal behaviour. It must be remembered that the fit is only a symptom of epilepsy, and one which may be absent or of slight importance in any given case. For this reason many individuals who are epileptic are not recognized as such, and the true cause of the delinquency which may develop, is overlooked. As an example of the epileptic delinquent, we may cite the case of a boy of fifteen, who got into trouble for staying out at night, and finally getting into a railway waggon and being carried off a hundred miles from his home. His mother had died when he was eight, his father had enlisted, and he had been sent to live with his grandmother. He had had some fits as a small child, but not since, though he was undoubtedly of the epileptic type. He really cared for no one but himself, and just did things he wanted to, coming and going just as he liked. During the year which had elapsed since leaving school, he had been in no less than six different jobs. He had gone to each with considerable enthusiasm, but had quickly tired of them after a week or two, and had just left his work undone. At the time he was seen, nothing would satisfy him but that he should join a regimental band and go out to India. The suggestion that he might be sorry to leave his relations or his brothers and sisters, seemed to fill him with considerable surprise, such a thing had never occurred to him.

Congenital syphilis may produce mental deficiency in all its degrees, but statistics show that it is not such a fruitful source of this as some think. However, apart from this, the interference with function of the more superficial layers of cortex may produce a cross-grained character, who may perpetrate the most bizarre acts and even dreadful crimes. For example, a child of three took pleasure in placing the kitten on the fire, and finally tried to grill his baby brother. This latter exploit persuaded the parents that it was time to seek medical advice, and in this case, treatment seems to have eradicated this cruel streak, and the child shows promise of growing up to be a decent citizen.

Encephalitis lethargica has been proved to have a considerable influence in changing the character of previously normal children. One child, after this disease, became sexually uncontrolled and quite without modesty. She insisted in disrobing in the middle of the street, and in making improper advances to any man she met. Another would brook no interference with his own desires and if any boy in the school crossed him he would fly at him, and fasten his teeth on any exposed part of his person. This boy had been backward before, but never vicious, the illness completed the mischief and the lower egocentric impulses became completely uncontrolled. There was an interesting development in this case, as some three years after the illness, when his conduct was becoming insupportable, it was found that he had never been punished. When this was suggested, the boy was most surprised and said "You can't punish me, I have had encephalitis lethargica." In spite of this ingenuous protest he was chastised, and for a time the effect was magical. Soon, however, it became obvious that the appeal was purely hedonistic, for the old impulses overcame his dread of pain, and the vicious behaviour re-established itself.

Shrubshall[5] has described a series of such cases, and showed that the character defects were similar to those associated with epilepsy—egocentricity and antisocial behaviour. Most people are agreed that the incidence of this disease is likely to result in a serious social problem in the future, a problem, indeed, with which we are all too unready to cope.

In order that a personality shall be integrated and controlled, the units of which the personality is composed must be present in certain proportions. If one or more of these are out of proportion to the rest, proper integration is impossible to achieve. Further, it would seem that these units must be arranged in certain ways and according to certain laws, so that they enter into these definite combinations which go to make up the normal personality. McDougall[6] and Shand[7] have shown what are the units from which the character is built, and how they are integrated together to form the sentiments, which are the major constituents of the human personality; and this integration, as it should proceed, has been sketched out. Difficulty may arise, because certain of the units are out of proportion to the rest, and also because the units combine in such a way that unusual emergents of behaviour result In the first case, we may find that fear, anger, sex, self-assertion, or any of the other units predominate to such an extent, that they come to overshadow the whole reaction of the child. The case in which almost every stimulus calls out fear, is not unfamiliar, and all efforts to teach the child to control this fear are largely unavailing, he remains the frightened, cowering, helpless being, from start to finish. The aggressive, quarrelsome child is also familiar and, though if physically strong he may hector his way through life more or less successfully from his own point of view, he is certainly difficult, if not delinquent. If he is physically weak, then he becomes spiteful and suspicious, seeks underhand ways of getting even with his real or fancied opponents, and may well drift into delinquency along this path. The child with too strongly developed sex is specially liable to come to grief, for society opposes to him little else than a string of negatives, and a series of bogeys. As a schoolmaster said of a set of school rules, there is no good in presenting to boys 150 "don'ts"; the weak boys are left with nothing to do, and the aggressive boys are merely instigated to do the things that are forbidden. One boy was asked what he thought of the rules of a school. He evidently had a poor opinion of them all, but he positively disliked rule 28, which forbade a boy to enter or leave the school by aeroplane, as he asked, what was the good of that? He couldn't even break it. Positive guidance is essential in the formation of character, and in respect of sex, this is conspicuously lacking in most systems of education.

In this connexion may be considered the precocious child, who becomes delinquent. This precocity may be intellectual or manipulative. In either case, the precocious ability will demand satisfaction and employment. If this is not obtained in the ordinary routine of school work, then some other scope must be found. If the precocity is intellectual, then it tends to express itself in phantasy, and if much of the child's intellectual activity is exercised in this phantasy, it may become very real and acquire a value little short of that felt for his normal surroundings. Such phantasy may find scope in early literary achievement, but is apt to expand itself merely on the dreaming of dreams. In any case, such activities are not likely to be very popular with the other children in the school, so that the youngster in question becomes more and more solitary, and often gets depressed and discouraged. Under these circumstances he finds refuge in his phantasies from the rebuffs of an unsympathetic world. Of such stuff are many truants made, and the truancy may vary from a deliberate avoidance of uncongenial surroundings, to a true fugue, in which the subject loses all touch with time and space, and is quite unaware afterwards where he has been or what he has done. The child in whom precocity is manifested in manipulation, is in better case under present conditions of school life, as he will usually find an outlet for his manual dexterity in some sort of game. In lower levels of society, however, this may not hold, and a child may only be able to find an outlet for his manipulative precocity in delinquency. For instance, the eight-year-old son of a law clerk noted for the excellence of his calligraphy, inherited a considerable degree of this manual dexterity. So precocious was he in this respect, that he soon achieved a reputation as the most expert pick-pocket in the Borough.

In the instances sketched above, stress has been laid on various causative influences which have been beyond conscious control, and have determined delinquencies, in spite of, rather than because of "deliberate choice." Many people will consider this one-sided, and think that a large proportion of delinquents deliberately choose this career for themselves, in the same way as another person would become a lawyer, a parson or a plumber. It is first necessary to define what is meant by deliberate choice. In this connexion Healey has defined the term as, "A choice made by those who possess mental powers sufficient for self-determination of the direction of their careers, in whom there are not—perforce of overpowering physical and mental characteristics—such internal tendencies as well might be calculated to develop criminalism, and in whom there is no overwhelming push from environmental sources." Distinction must then be drawn in the study of the delinquent personality, between the criminal who chooses crime on the first occasion, and the boy who becomes a habitual and professional criminal because social conditions have prevented him taking up any desirable occupation. He is a criminal of necessity, and not of choice, if we remember that the feebleness of his own character prevents him succeeding along legitimate lines, and so may constitute a large part of the necessity. As Healey says, "I should insist, that if deliberate choice is to be invoked by way of explanation of an antisocial career, there must have been plenty of opportunity, and even invitation, to take advantage of occupational or recreational interests, which would have proved enticing enough to cause others to choose refraining from misdeeds. Narrowed down in this way, it would seem, that the adoption of criminality as a career from deliberate choice is exceedingly rare." To quote Healey again, "Making up our minds at many different times, and often in consultation with experienced people and with the great amount of material which often has been collected on a case, it is significant that we find justification for applying the phrase 'deliberate choice' as a cause, in less than half a dozen instances, in more than 1000 cases of repeated offenders." A study of these six cases, however, shows an abnormal personality, lacking balance between the hereditary disposition, or a more than usual capacity for being influenced by a hostile environment. It may be concluded, therefore, that in the same way as with so many other types of human behaviour, crime is determined by the influence of affectively toned "wishes"; but that where the level of consciousness is reached at which organization is sufficient to allow for discrimination and control, deliberate antisocial behaviour is unusual.

These considerations may to some extent serve to answer the question: why is the child like this? To answer the question as to what we must do with the child, the answer is that we must do one of two things or both, we must alter the child, or we must alter the environment. One thing must be made quite clear. The apologists for the delinquent child must have no desire to dictate to schoolmasters or justices, or suggest for a moment that they should change the methods which their experience has shown to work well. The duty of the schoolmaster and the judge is to the majority, that is to the normal child and to society as a whole, and if the delinquent child is a misfit, he may have to be removed, and it may be to his advantage to be removed. Schools are being started here and there, which specialize in taking misfits. If these are run by the right people and are kept small, they may be a great success and should be multiplied. Where circumstances permit, individual tuition may be very desirable for a time, for by this means the real capacity of the child can be determined. He may require greater intellectual outlet, or he may require greater manipulative opportunity. The development of more experimental work in the schools is undoubtedly useful. The more a child can work out and do for himself, the better it gives him confidence and a sense of power over his environment which is essentially healthy. In the lower walks of life, the industrial school or the training ship are the usual goal of the delinquent child. In these institutions the discipline and opportunity of achievement, work wonders for the majority, but it must be recognized that a few never fit in, while others drift back as soon as they are once more put on their own resources. This only means, that like other human institutions, these methods are not perfect; and by greater knowledge and fuller understanding, efforts must be made to improve them further.

The other approach to the problem is to change the child, and to do this we must change his outlook on life. Before this can be accomplished we must discover what this outlook is, and if we are to understand this, we must put aside all "sensible" adult preconceptions. The mind of the child is very different from that of the adult, and his outlook is often extraordinarily disproportionate and limited. He must be made to understand the real truth, be encouraged to present his difficulties, which must be dealt with calmly and unemotionally. If we are to help him, we must never show ourselves shocked, or surprised, or amused, however extravagant his ideas, or perverted his actions.

In dealing with children who have started on a life of crime, it is striking how uniform is the delinquency but how diverse the personality. As R. C. Cabot remarks, "How diverse the virtues! how similar the crimes! Is it not amazing,—the smooth uniformity of nail-biting, bunking out, truancy, obscenity and theft? In these elements the stories are so much alike that one almost forgets which is which, until the child himself speaks up. . . . Perhaps each sin, as the sinner and God see it, is as unique as any part of his personality. But certain it is that the records of delinquency, as the world's coarse thumb and finger sort them out in piles, obscure the clear outlines of the children till they look unnaturally, untruly alike." Every delinquent is an individual, a new emergent owing something to heredity, something to environment, and something to the adaptation between these, but always a new personality, for which none of these alone can be said to be responsible

Moreover the more complete the investigation, the more complicated is the record of potential or actual delinquencies, a child is seldom found to be only a thief, or only a truant, or what not; other abnormalities are revealed, and all are due to the lack of balance and control in the personality. For instance, many of the cases of theft in children are a great puzzle. Occasionally such thefts may be merely the result of uncontrolled acquisitive instinct, but often this is only uncontrolled because it is reinforced by some other impulses. For example, a girl who was the daughter of a vain pleasure-loving woman, was adopted by a virtuous but severe spinster who denied her all personal adornments. When the child went to school, she began to steal small sums of money, which were all spent on cheap jewelry and ribbons. With these she adorned herself in secret, to her great gratification. This problem was never investigated, but it is not improbable that had she been permitted some personal decoration, and been taught to keep this within reasonable limits rather than to repress it altogether, there might have been no theft. Again, a girl stole money from the mistresses but spent it all on sweets which she gave to other girls. The feeling of inferiority and desire to please her class-mates which underlay this delinquency, is obvious. Cases of stealing from the parents are frequent in the juvenile courts, and in many of these it is clear that the theft is instigated by a desire to get even with the parent, or often with a step-parent, for some real or fancied grievance. A strong feeling of protest against society is often the basis of a career of crime, and if a child's lot in the home, or in society could be alleviated, much that is criminal might be avoided. So we must conclude that the delinquent personality is an unbalanced personality, and like all unbalanced persons, requires individual study, for without this we can never know what particular factor is responsible for the deviation from the mean which determines his failure in adaptation. Moreover, these studies contribute to our general store of knowledge of personality, for which of us is not tempted to gratify our own wishes in ways contrary to the decalogue? Though we may rejoice when the wicked are punished, if we be truly honest, we must murmur to ourselves, as the prisoner is removed to his cell, "there, but for the grace of God, go I." Indeed, those who attempt to do social work amongst the criminal classes will never be truly successful, unless they are brave enough, to admit this truth fully.

CHAPTER XV

THE DISSOCIATED PERSONALITY

In the study of the psychological integration of the personality, attention was drawn to the constitution of the sentiments, with the self-regarding sentiment as the dominant and controlling influence. These sentiments may, or may not be permanent, and may wax and wane, according to changed circumstances in the environment. A sentiment has been defined as the organization of a series of dispositions in relation to an object, and the best examples of sentiments are those of love and hate. The organization in the case of love is so constituted that the object of the sentiment is continually benefited by the resulting behaviour. On the other hand, in the case of hate all behaviour is to the detriment of the object. From the teleological standpoint, therefore, these two sentiments are diametrically opposed. Yet, according to the principle of ambivalence of the emotions, enunciated by Freud and referred to in Chapter IX, the same object may be loved and hated alternately; indeed, it would seem that in some cases the two sentiments were in operation almost coincidently. Again it is a familiar observation that the object of a sentiment of love or hate may change with bewildering rapidity with some people, so that they are on with the new love almost before they are off with the old. Thus it is evident, that not only may the group of emotional dispositions, organized in relation to an object, rapidly change, but also the object may change in relation to the emotional disposition. The dissociated personality exemplifies this mutability of the sentiments in an exaggerated degree, but a study of such personalities serves to illustrate an important feature in the normal. For example, consider the possibilities of dissociation within the self-regarding sentiment, which is the organization of the emotional dispositions in relation to the ego and its reactions with the environment. This sentiment is a late development as McDougall[1] points out, for "the conception of a self must have reference to other selves"; it is only by comparison with other beings that the ego can be appreciated as a unity different from the rest. Consequently, like all recently acquired functions, it tends to be instable and easily modified. Further this self-regarding sentiment largely depends for its constitution on the experiences which have been enjoyed in the past, as Prince[2] has pointed out, both in respect to their influence in moulding the ego, and in so far as the ego makes reflective judgments on these experiences.

Amongst the other emotional dispositions organized in this sentiment, those of self-abasement and self-assertion are of great importance. One or other of these will always be dominant and the degree of success in the adaptation of the individual to the environment will determine, at any given moment, which of these is the ascendant. If adaptation is successful, then self-assertion will tend to be prominent, while if the reverse be the case, self-abasement will govern the nature of the sentiment. It is clear that the success of adaptation of any individual varies from time to time according to the nature of the environment in which he finds himself, and this variation is accompanied by modification in his self-regarding sentiment. Such variations may be more or less persistent and may be classed as moods. They are exemplified by the alternating states of exultation and depression, or of interest and apathy, which are met with in their extreme form in psychopathic personalities, and in less regular forms in the normal. The recovering neurotic shows this alternation very clearly. On his good days, when he has achieved adaptation, he is confident that he can do anything, that he is quite well and will never be ill any more. Perhaps the next day he feels bad, something has happened to upset his adaptation and his attitude is entirely different, he can do nothing, he is more ill than anyone has ever been before, and he will never get well. There is more here than a mere change of mood, or variation in temperament; the same man on the two consecutive days is a totally different personality, and were it not for his bodily features remaining the same, he might be regarded as two separate individuals. To a lesser degree, this change in the self-regarding sentiment, with its accompanying change in personality, occurs in day dreams and dreams proper. In the dream, dispositions take on a new organization within the ego, perhaps to such an extent, that, as Plato says, the good man dreams what the bad man does. In the dream, the normally good man becomes a bad man, the coward becomes a hero, or the reverse may happen and the normally brave man becomes a coward. Such dreams may either be prospective or retrospective. In his studies of dream analysis Jung[3] has laid stress on the former type, while Freud[4] has concentrated on the latter. In the former case, such as the dream in which the coward becomes a hero, there is a fulfilment in phantasy of the aspirations of the individual towards something higher than himself, to which he is struggling in his life and which he has not yet, and perhaps never will reach. In the latter type there is a fulfilment of wishes belonging to the primitive instincts, and in the phantasy they escape from the fetters of higher controls and integrations active in waking life. Such low level impulses are the normal directive agents of the bad man's character, and hence the truth of Plato's aphorism. Dissociations between phantasy and real behaviour are common in the experience of the ordinary man. Indeed, if we consider it from this point of view, we are all liable to become multiple personalities when the higher integration and control are in abeyance during sleep. Our self-regarding sentiment becomes dominated, now by self-assertion, now by self-abasement, now by fear, now by anger and so on, and with each dream-variant we assume a new rôle in life's drama. As a general rule, such dreams only involve ideational and affective activity, and no overt action takes place, but in some cases complex activity may be observed In these cases so-called somnambulistic states arise, and actions of a complicated nature may be performed. Such activities are the result of a change of attitude of the ego to the environment, and the dominance of the self-regarding sentiment, not by a simple emotion, but by a subsidiary sentiment. Frequently this change is of the nature of a regression, so that the individual is attempting an adjustment to an experience or an environment which has long since passed away. This will be accompanied by a special arrangement of emotional dispositions, suitable to the past experience, but unsuited to the present, which may take the form of a mood of excitement, elation or depression, by a series of images and ideas relating to the experience which has passed, and by a series of actions which are illustrative or symbolic of this experience. For example, on returning from the war a man developed "attacks" during which he lost all touch with his surroundings. If they occurred during the day-time, he would be unaware what he was doing or where he was going. Yet all the time he would walk along without stumbling. In other words, his habitual automatic actions were performed adequately, but his attention was directed elsewhere. During the attack he experienced fear and anxiety, and "expressed" these feelings in his general appearance. At the same time, he performed various gestures which were inexplicable, both to himself and to his companions. Later, it was possible to discover that during these "attacks" he was paying attention to a series of images which were accompanied by emotional experience and certain gestures appropriate to them. These images represented himself and his mother serving a company in a menial capacity. The host and hostess of this company were a banker and his daughter. To this daughter he had at one time been much attached, but monetary losses had resulted in a change in his social sphere which made marriage impossible. As a rule, this set of ideas was seldom, if ever, in his mind, since he had done his best to repress it and dissociate it. That is to say, the group of emotional dispositions organized round his conception of himself in relation to his environment did not usually include this other subsidiary sentiment of love for the banker's daughter. But with a change in the orientation of the self-regarding sentiment, this love sentiment became dominant, to the exclusion of every other subsidiary sentiment. To put the state of affairs in another way, as a rule the general organization of his mental activities was towards his present recovery from the effects of the war, and his future means of livelihood. Suddenly, he would regress to a former state, in which the organization of his mental activities was towards marriage with the banker's daughter. Yet this regression was not complete for, in the phantasy, he and his mother appeared in a menial capacity, and not as equals, and the fulfilment of his wish seemed impossible. A similar state is met with in the person who falls into a "brown study," but in this case there is little or no amnesia as to the sentiment dominant during the phase. In the case quoted above there was no vivid recollection of the mental content of the attack, until revived by special psychotherapeutic measures. The state of affairs in the "brown study" clearly depends on inhibition. Just as the action of the extensor muscles is inhibited while a limb is being flexed, just as the whole emotional disposition of fear may be inhibited while a cat goes to the rescue of her kittens who are in danger, so, at a higher level, one group of subordinate sentiments in the self-regarding sentiment, are inhibited during the dominance of another group. Under other circumstances, the latter group may be inhibited and the former dominant. This inhibition may be purely transient, as in the case of a mood, when affect is chiefly involved in the inhibited and dominant pattern, or again in the "brown study." Or the inhibition may be permanent, in the case of somnambulisms, which usually chiefly involve ideational patterns, or in states of depression or exultation, when affective patterns are involved. This alternating inhibition is what is known as dissociation, and the importance of the patterns dissociated, within the self-regarding sentiment, vary considerably. In the case quoted above, the dissociated pattern involving the sentiment of love for the banker's daughter was not an essential part of the patient's present make-up, and its temporary dominance did not involve any marked change in the patient's life and general behaviour. In other cases, however, the degree of importance of dissociated patterns is of great variety. Janet[5] has described these cases with great detail and lucidity. The simple cases, such as the one quoted, he calls monoideistic somnambulisms. These involve the dominance of a pattern relating to one scene, event, or object, though in themselves, such patterns may be very complex. "One of the characteristics of these somnambulisms is that they repeat themselves indefinitely. Not only are the different attacks always exactly alike, repeating the same movements, expressions and words, but in the course of the same attack, when it has lasted a certain time, the same scene may be repeated again in exactly the same way, five or ten times. At last, the agitation seems to wear out, the dream grows less clear, and gradually or suddenly according to the case, the patient comes back to her normal consciousness, takes up her ordinary business, quite undisturbed by what has happened." In other words, the rest of the sentiments and patterns inhibited during the attack, again become dominant, and the previously dominant pattern becomes inhibited. If these changes are sudden, they are sometimes accompanied by a severe pain in the head. What physical change this corresponds to is not certain, but there must be a profound change in the synaptial junctions to induce the sudden inhibitions of large engraphic patterns. Such biochemical changes may well be accompanied by vascular or other modifications, such as might induce severe pain. In the case of the monoideistic somnambulisms, the whole proceeding is apt to be carried out with great intensity and vehemence. This is characteristic of those patterns of behaviour of a relatively simple nature, uncontrolled by the other patterns, which make up the total mental constituents.

In the next group of cases, described by Janet as polyideistic somnambulisms, or fugues, there is no real difference, but the dissociated pattern is much more complex and comprehensive. Here the temporarily dominant abnormal pattern governs the conduct of the individual for days or months together, and may lead to a wandering away, so that he finds himself far from his home, without any conception as to how he got there. For example, a lady became very depressed and convinced of her own inadequacy, both to manage her own household and to attend to her religious duties. While she was in this mood, she suddenly lost touch with her surroundings and started to walk away. She had only a few pence in her pocket, and these she spent on some buns in a baker's shop. Finally she "came to herself" in a village ten miles from home, in a very fatigued and foot-sore condition. She had no knowlege of how she got there nor what she had done in the interval, and it was only afterwards, that the story of her walk and of the purchase of the buns was elicited. Such is a very simple fugue, but many of those described in literature are of great complexity and duration. They differ from the simpler somnabulisms, not only in their greater complexity, but also in the fact that the behaviour involved is of less intensity and violence. This is due to the fact that the pattern which becomes dominant is more complex and fully integrated, and so the activation of more numerous neurones belonging to a higher level is involved. The more neurones involved in the production of any pattern of behaviour, the less intense and violent will be that behaviour. It has already been pointed out, that the explanation of this lies in the resistance offered at the synaptial junctions to the spread of activation. It may be, that in these complicated alternations of character it would be better to express the change as one of orientation of the various affective and conative combinations within the self-regarding sentiment, rather than the dominance of an entirely separate pattern, which would suppose the activation of a quite separate group of neurones. Hence the change might be more adequately expressed, by supposing the activation to flow over a different course amongst the neurones, and thus produce a new engram, though many of the actual neurones involved in the production of the rival patterns are the same. This is specially so with the next group of cases, those of double personality. In these, the individual alternately presents two or more states, in which the personality differs profoundly. It sometimes happens that there is a complete amnesia for one state when the person is in the other; but often the condition, to which Morton Prince has given the name co-consciousness, is met with. In this there is complete awareness of the other state, through which the individual has passed. Discussion of such cases is out of place here, since they are very rare, and good accounts of the classical examples may be found in literature, while Dr Morton Prince's description of Miss Beauchamp, in his *Dissociation of a Personality*,[6] is now familiar to most people interested in the subject.

The reference to the subject of dissociated personality serves to correct the impression that there is a complete and perfect integration of sentiment in the normal individual, and to show how, not only may one or more sentiments be divorced from the rest without losing their power of influencing behaviour, or waning altogether, but also, that new orientations may arise within the more complex sentiments, so that the whole attitude and adaptation of the individual becomes profoundly altered.[7] This alteration of attitude may be described as another example of instability, and this is certainly the case, but there can be no harm in insisting on the fact that at the present stage of evolution, stability of integration is not characteristic of the average personality, and that it is in this direction of fuller integration, that we may look for further advance and the emergence of that quality of deity, promised to us by Alexander.[8]

It is probable that the change of orientation within the sentiment is, at any rate partly, a product of endocrine activity influencing the biochemical balance at the synaptial junctions. Such activities may be induced through the blood stream, by what would be termed physical influences, such as fatigue products, poisons, etc., or may be induced by way of the central and sympathetic nervous systems, by what may be termed psychic influences, such as perceptions and images. The great difficulty in any such theory of action is of course to explain why an endocrine change, which presumably reaches all the synapses by way of the blood and cerebro-spinal fluid, should cause inhibition of one group and facilitation of another. Our only answer can be that we do not know. Yet it is quite clearly established in physiology that selective inhibition and facilitation do occur, as for instance in the simultaneous contractions of the body, and relaxation of the neck of hollow viscera. Also Pharmacology teaches us that such drugs as curare, strychnine, etc., have a very specific action on certain very limited structures in the nervous system, and the analogy which we seek to draw does not seem impossibly far-fetched.

It is clear that such alterations as orientation within the sentiments are absolutaly necessary in everyday life, in order that we may adapt ourselves to the ever varying circumstances of our environment; and it seems quite possible that the pathological examples, such as have been quoted, represent that little more, which nature so often displays, and which makes the difference between health and disease.

CHAPTER XVI

THE RETARDED PERSONALITY

MENTION has already been made of the difficulty in estimating the stages of evolutionary development leading up to the emergence of consciousness, with the development of complete cortical function. In the normal child, the stages are passed through so quickly, and at a time when so little corroboration can be obtained from the object of our study, that little help can be got in establishing a clear picture of the process. In the retarded personality, however, it is possible to obtain a little more indication. In this case, mental growth takes place to a certain point and then stops, as the development of the cortex is arrested, so that some sort of picture is presented, which may be studied at leisure. Even so, however, the problem is not so simple as it might at first sight appear, since cortical function is so complex that the retardation is not necessarily universal in its incidence; as, for example, in those cases referred to in Chapter XIV, in whom intellectual development and control is good, but the control of the affective reactions is deficient. Further bodily development, so far as it comprises structures outside the central nervous system, may proceed normally, and we have already seen the effect of bodily, and especially endocrine activity on mental process. Hence it is obvious that we must not regard the mental reactions of a cortex which has stopped development at the stage of a child of five, when it is under the influence of adult thyroid and sex gland function, as identical with the normal condition of a child of this age, when the cortical function should be under the influence of thymus and juvenile thyroid function.

Necessarily, retardation of personality implies some degree of mental deficiency, but for the purposes of the present discussion it is not desirable to regard the retarded personality and the mental deficient as exactly synonymous terms, otherwise some confusion might ensue. Tredgold[1] has classified mentally deficient children into two groups, of Primary Amentia and Secondary Amentia. The first, which comprises eighty per cent. of such cases, are the true retarded personalities, whose deficiency is due to some inherent defect, as a result of which full development of the personality is impossible. The second group comprises those who are defective as the result of inflammatory or degenerative processes, due to external causes. With these it is not proposed to deal at all, as the incidence of defect is liable to be much more complicated and irregular.

In order to establish the fact that there is some degree of retardation of the personality, it is necessary to have a standard whereby a normal may be established. Such a standard is not easy to come by, for it is abundantly clear that there must be great differences between personalities, and that while one may excel in one direction, he may lamentably fail in another. Spearman[2] and his followers have attempted to establish the existence of general intelligence factors which may be determined for any individual and compared with those of his neighbour, but their results have not been altogether convincing, and there are many who doubt the utility of estimating any such factor. However, some such standardization has been made possible by the work of Binet,[3] Simon, Terman,[4] Yerkes and others, who have elaborated a scale of tests whereby the mental age of any individual may be determined. By the term mental age is meant that the child tested reaches a standard commensurate with the general mental capacity of a normal child of such and such an age. Thus, a child of sixteen may only be able to respond accurately to tests suitable to a normal child of ten. We express this by saying that the child of actual age sixteen, has a mental age of ten. These tests are formulated with the idea of estimating the general inherent mental capacity, rather than the store of acquired knowledge. The acquisition of knowledge is quite a different thing from the power of application. This is shown very clearly in the case of certain Orientals. For example, in medical examinations it is frequently found that these people can do wonderfully well in the written papers, where they have an opportunity of presenting their acquired knowledge. When, however, they are taken to the wards and put before the case of a disease which they have discussed with the greatest glibness in the written papers, they are utterly at a loss and cannot apply their knowledge to practical issues. This practical application and ability to adapt to new requirements is essential to successful work in any sphere of life, hence it is clear that the tests must be directed to estimate these latter factors, and not mere general knowledge, if we are to assess the intellectual capacity of the subject. On these criteria, Terman stated that the mental age of twenty is the upper limit of intelligence, and that the average intelligence corresponds to the mental age sixteen. The wholesale tests carried out on the American army showed, however, that there are many people who do not reach the mental age of sixteen, but who are reasonably successful in adapting themselves to life; and it is usual to regard as definitely retarded, only those below the mental age of twelve. This is found to be the limit, below which it is impossible for the individual to maintain himself in the world and carry on his existence as an independent person, at a reasonable standard. It is the high grade mentally deficient mother who makes the slum out of even decent houses, and if we are to remove slums, we must provide better opportunities in the shape of enough houses first; but, unless we can improve the general mental capacity of the lower strata of society, our housing schemes will be largely unavailing.

At the lowest levels are those who, as James says, are nonplussed by all but the very simplest situations. These may never be capable of walking, talking or controlling their functions: and such cases who fall below the standard expected of the normal child of two are technically termed idiots. Those whose mental age is between three and seven are termed imbeciles, and in America those between seven and eleven are termed morons, a useful term which is finding considerable acceptance in this country. According to the English Mental Deficiency Act of 1913:

An Idiot is a person so deeply defective in mind as to be unable to guard himself against common physical dangers.

An Imbecile is a person in whose case there exists a mental defectiveness not amounting to idiocy: yet it is so pronounced that he is incapable of managing or being taught to manage himself or his affairs.

S

A Feeble-minded person is one in whom the mental defectiveness is so pronounced that he requires care, supervision and control, for his own protection or that of others ; or, in the case of a child, that he, by reason of such defectiveness, appears to be permanently incapable of receiving proper benefit from the instruction in ordinary schools.

The classification of retarded personalities is not an altogether simple matter, and in certain respects, the above-mentioned tests are misleading. In any given test, the achievement of the child may fall far short of his capacity, and in testing a suspected defective, consideration should always be given to various factors. Firstly, the child should be physically well, for apart from the malaise induced by physical disease, the sensations of discomfort, derived from the enteroceptors in the various organs absorb a considerable proportion of the child's attention and, if full attention cannot be given to the tests he cannot acquit himself as he should. Similarly, the test should be undertaken in a quiet place, free from outer distractions, so that the attention be not absorbed by extraneous sensations received through the exteroceptors. Thirdly, the full confidence of the child should be obtained, for nervousness and shyness will prevent his answering in accordance with his real capacity. Fourthly, if, as the result of the test, he fails to reach his proper age standard, care must be exercised to discover whether this apparent deficiency is due to a true general retardation, or to some repression and instability, such as is described in relation to the neurotic personality. Fifthly, one examination of a child does not determine the degree of deficiency, for retardation is by no means a sudden process, and there is generally a more or less gradual slowing down of normal development. Thus, a child may be apparently normal up to the age of five, then gradually fall behind his contemporaries, until he comes to a complete stop at the mental age of ten. To estimate this gradual retardation, it is clear that at least two tests, and preferably a series of tests spread over a period of time, are necessary.

Retardation of personality is associated and commensurate with a failure of complete development of the central nervous system, and especially of the cortex. However, even low grade imbeciles and idiots may present a brain, which in naked eye appearances differs little from that of the normal man. It is in the microscopic characters, and possibly in the biochemical composition of the cells and synapses, that marked changes are to be met with, and these defects show special incidence on the frontal region, and in the parietal association areas—the latest evolutionary developments. The characteristic differences of behaviour and capacity in the retarded personality correspond largely to the failure of proper functions which are associated with complete cortical development, namely integration, control, discrimination and localization. Even in the realm of motor activity these failures of control and integration are frequently noticeable, for many defectives exhibit purposeless involuntary movements of the limbs, and facial grimaces which are characteristic of uncontrolled subcortical motor activity. Such movements are more or less normal in the young infant, in whom the full control of the motor cortex has not yet been established; and indeed, it is only gradually and at different intervals, that the full control of the various functions is arrived at. The development of this control can be studied in the growing child, but there is such constant development and change that the study is one of great difficulty; but the static condition of the retarded personality gives us a series of pictures which may be compared to the slow motion pictures in the cinematograph, allowing us to study complicated movements in greater detail.

Since we are dealing with personality as met with in the so-called normal, the lower forms of mental defect, such as idiocy and imbecility, have much less interest for us as a whole. Yet they do illustrate arrests at levels which represent infantile behaviour. The idiot often shows marked sensory defects, deafness and blindness being not uncommon accompaniments. Skin anæsthesias are also relatively common, some idiots being able to tolerate transfixion of the skin with pins, without experiencing pain. Apart from the actual presence of the sensation, perception is markedly deficient or totally absent, the idiot sees but does not look, hears but does not listen, and feels touch and pain but does not refer them in space and time.

The emotional dispositions are not developed, and the idiot does not rise much above the more complex reflexes, such as crying when hurt. There is no voluntary control of the bladder and bowel, and these organs empty reflexly. Similarly food is masticated and swallowed if placed in the mouth, but there is no effort to seek for food and if not fed, the idiot would starve. Like very young children, he often sleeps a great deal, but may be restless and fretful.

The imbecile takes an intermediate position between the almost entirely reflex idiot, and the feeble-minded, about to be described, and reacts largely on the basis of his emotional dispositions.

Among the feeble-minded we have illustrations of arrests at levels to which many so-called normals may sink under the influences of sickness, or other adversities, and from which some do not raise themselves very far. It is worth while, therefore, to survey briefly the nature of various mental functions in such cases. It will be remembered that the engraphic patterns in the nervous system are primarily inherent, that is definitely "set" at birth, so that specific stimuli are followed by specific actions. These may retain their primary arrangements more or less throughout life, or the "set" of the pattern is markedly modified by contact with the environment, and this contact establishes new combinations of neurones to form new patterns. These patterns of neurones, when thrown into activity, have for their mental aspect various mental processes and patterns of behaviour. As would be expected from the concept of retardation, the inherent patterns show little modification, but the feeble-minded are deficient in acquired modifications. This is because their nervous system is relatively poor in neurones, and is therefore incapable of responding to the innumerable fresh stimuli which crowd in upon the child after birth, and increase in number and variety with every month of life. At the same time, and for the same reason, the modes of action are restricted, and so activity in these people tends to be stereotyped and lacking in agility and adaptation. The moron's greatest difficulty is in meeting new situations, and while the same task may be performed over and over again, so long as there is no change in the circumstances, yet, if a new situation arises, no new adaptation follows. Similarly with speech, a few stock phrases suffice for most purposes, and there is no possibility of adorning a tale, or explaining a situation, by a varied flow of language. It is a well-known fact that the feeble-minded sometimes have an amazingly retentive memory, so that they can reproduce whole pages by rote. Varendonck[5] has distinguished between what he calls reduplicative memory and synthetical memory. By the first he means a recall of a series of associated ideas and sensations, in their exact chronological and spatial order, without discrimination or selection. By the latter he means the selective recall of certain significant units out of a series of associations, from which arises perception and the attachment of meaning. The feeble-minded excel in the former type of memory, and Varendonck has shown how this reduplicative memory may be quite independent of consciousness. It would appear that this type of memory depends on a series of stimuli producing an engraphic effect on a comparatively simple series of neurones, without that widespread activation which involves the cortical function of discrimination and selection. The reactivation of the engram resulting from stimuli, is therefore followed by an exact reproduction, which is so characteristic of the more feeble-minded even in ordinary life, as, for example, two garrulous old women gossiping on their door-step.

This also explains why interruption by an ill-timed question in the middle of the discourse, often necessitates recommencement from the beginning. For there is no power of discrimination, and very often, little appreciation of the meaning of what is being said. Persons of low grade intelligence frequently find employment as guides in historic buildings, and reel off again and again, to successive parties, long discourses involving a wealth of historical detail, with appropriate dates and names. This sometimes gives the impression of deep erudition, until the guide is asked intelligent questions, when he gazes with blank amazement at his interlocutor, and is unable to appreciate even what the question means.

Similarly, when we study the powers of association in the feeble-minded, we find that they have considerable facility for association by contiguity, when a series of stimuli directly impress a series of neurone patterns so as to form a simple engram. Association by similarity however, is poor, for in such cases a much wider range of experience is required, with the consequent great complication of the engrams. A further light on this is to be found with reference to the "Gestalt" theory. Perception is not merely a summation of sensations associated with images, but is a new emergent, or, as the Gestalt theory would express it, a structural totality, which must exist before meaning can arise and consciousness of the object exist. Köhler,[6] in his experiments on the anthropoid, has shown that apes are capable of experiencing such totalities, but that these are relatively limited and simple. Similarly, the feeble-minded can only experience limited and simple "Gestalten." As a result of the limitation of these higher emergents, their perceptions are limited, and, owing to dearth of material, their power of discriminating and comparing is poor. It follows, therefore, that associations by similarity are deficient, for the simplicity of the "Gestalten" is in accordance with association by contiguity. This brings us back to our starting point, that the higher cortical function is deficient.

For the same reason, the power of integrating and organizing the various perceptions is lacking, and so, no well organized complex engrams easily emerge. On the contrary, a series of simple disconnected engrams are constantly being activated, with the result that the controlled organized activation which involves attention is not attained easily. Hence, the feeble-minded are found to have difficulty in fixing and holding their attention on one definite object; they flit from one thing to another, as activation passes from one engram to another. This deficiency in the more comprehensive structural patterns, and in the power of fixing attention, necessarily results in difficulty of smooth adaptation to new surroundings or events. For, in order to achieve this smooth adaptation, a definite connexion between the events must be appreciated.

Failure of adaptation applies equally to the physical and mental processes, so that just as retarded persons cannot adapt their bodily movements to new occupations, so they cannot adapt their minds to new situations. They show, therefore, a marked deficiency in the power of creative imagination. By this is meant, the power of perceiving new relationships, so that a new mental emergent results. They cannot invent or improvise. Since wit and humour depend, to a large extent, on creative imagination, their attempts at humour are of the silliest type, and their appreciation of it is of the most crude and elementary description.

On the affective side of mental life, the moron experiences the primary emotions in the normal way; indeed, in view of the general want of control, he may react more violently than does the normal person. This may easily be seen in the case of fear or anger. He is specially prone to panics and rages. At the same time, there is a want of discrimination and modification both of stimuli and reactions. Thus, in the case of fear, any danger, whether remote or imminent, is likely to produce much the same degree of emotional reaction, and there is little power of learning by experience to neglect certain stimuli which appear frightening but are in reality harmless; or conversely, to avoid stimuli which appear harmless but are in reality noxious. Similarly with the reaction to the stimulus. The normal person learns to adopt a reaction which is most suitable to the particular stimulus pattern of the moment. The feeble-minded will not modify his reaction, but always tends to follow the same behaviour. For example, a boy of low intelligence had been in the habit of hiding his head in response to noises which frightened him. In course of time he was enlisted, and had to go to the war. One day, he was in a building which was struck by a shell. After the confusion had subsided, he was found with his head in the bread sack! The same habitual reaction was to him the right one, whatever the danger. The organization of these primitive simple emotions into the more complex emotional reactions is always poor and the defective never experiences the more complex emotions such as awe or reverence. McDougall[7] has described awe as an integration of fear, self-abasement and curiosity; and it is certainly the case that the feeble-minded child does not develop awe for anything. Yet, he is certainly not without the three primary emotions which comprise it. Nor are these entirely without integration. For example, in one case who came under observation because she got into difficulties, it was found that the abnormal behaviour depended very largely on the three above-mentioned primary emotions. In her case, her attitude towards events was a sort of sly approach, which cannot be expressed by any one term. This involved a certain integration of fear, curiosity and self-abasement. The emergent, however, was of a decidedly lower quality than awe, because the relatedness was different, and of a less high order. For the same reason, and to a greater degree, the feeble-minded are deficient in the highly organized sentiments, and except for routine habitual action, are never able to stick at one thing long if it involves any effort of adaptation. For example, they may love, but there is little discrimination in their love, and they either love every one, or hate every one; nor is the love particularly selfless, but depends rather on benefits received.

It is in wisely directed habit formation that the salvation of the retarded personality lies, for habit involves simple neurone patterns. It must be remembered, however, that, as James[8] points out, habits are of two kinds. The impulsive habit is a direct expression of an unimpeded impulse, such as that cited above of the boy who always hid his head at the threat of danger. As these are not as a rule adapted to the requirements of varying circumstances, and are usually egocentric, they are almost always bad habits. The moron is very liable to such habits, owing to the lack of discrimination and control which characterizes all his behaviour, and in training these people such habit formation has to be avoided most carefully. The so-called voluntary habit is, however, a different matter, and consists of a mode of behaviour which has been founded on foresight and discrimination. Although the feeble-minded is incapable of exercising that foresight and discrimination for himself, there is no reason why others should not do it for him; and indeed, these habits are easily established. It stands to reason that the foresight may be directed towards evil ends as well as good; and that is why it is so important to protect the retarded personality from those who would use him for their own purposes.

It is unnecessary to elaborate the fact that the feeble-minded is incapable of the higher intellectual processes of judgment and reasoning, since these require the discrimination between well-organized patterns, in which he is conspicuously lacking. Similarly, he is always weak willed. Voluntary action involves decision between two opposing possibilities. This decision depends on a rapid and concise organization of all the stimuli, both exteroceptive and proprioceptive, pertaining to one possibility, with the images involving previous related experiences, so that this "outweighs" the other possibility, and appropriate muscular activation ensues accordingly. Such prompt and definite integration is impossible for the moron, so that he is vacillating and uncertain, constantly pulled this way and that, as one ill-organized pattern momentarily gains ascendancy.

Such are the reactions of the retarded personality, an all too familiar member of our community. Call to mind Millet's picture of the "Man with the Hoe," and Markham's words:

> "Bowed by the weight of centuries he leans,
> Upon his hoe, and gazes on the ground,
> The emptiness of ages in his face
> And on his back, the burden of the world.
> Who made him dead to rapture and despair,
> A thing that grieves not and that never hopes,
> Stolid and stunned, a brother to the ox?
> Who loosened and let down that brutal jaw?"

For our purpose of understanding personality, the study of the feeble-minded affords us several data. As has been said, we can study in a more or less static form various phases in the development of the normal adult. We can appreciate what is the result from the psychical aspect of a failure of complete development of brain structure. We can recognize how the consequent failure of psychical elaboration and integration determines and restricts behaviour. Finally, we can realize how this limitation in potential reaction with the environment impoverishes the total personality.

CHAPTER XVII

THE SPIRITUAL ASPECT OF PERSONALITY

MANY people regard the physiological approach to the study of Personality with distaste, because to them it seems that it is entirely materialistic, and forbids any looking forward or any purpose in life. It would seem quite certain that some sort of spiritual outlook is essentially a human characteristic, and is inevitable, once self-consciousness and reflective thought have emerged as new entities in the march of evolution. Moreover, some sort of philosophy of life is absolutely necessary, if the personality is to be properly organized and enabled to get through life. One of the most characteristic features of the maladapted neurotic is that he is not provided, in many cases, with an adequate philosophy of life. The phrase philosophy of life is used in preference to religion, because a religion may be professed by certain people, without their acquiring thereby any adequate working scheme to afford them an explanation of their true relationship with the environment and with the universe as a whole. This is not to say that religion in its various forms does not serve many personalities as a perfectly adequate, and indeed, for them, the only possible philosophy. The purpose of this chapter must be therefore to inquire whether the personality, as sketched out, can have a spiritual aspect, and whether, from a psycho-physical standpoint, an adequate philosophy of life is conceivable. It must be understood that such a function of the personality is only possible at the highest level of evolution so far reached. Clearly, one of the chief functions which characterizes advance in mental power, is that of distinguishing the self from the environment. The development of this function can be observed in the young infant, who, at first, has no consciousness beyond the satisfaction of his various organic needs, and cannot distinguish his hands or feet from the objects around him. However, he gradually learns, as the result of his early experiences, that certain objects which he sees and feels are part of himself. From this gradually grows the realization that his own ego, both in respect of body and mind, is distinct from other egos and from the universe around him. Some have declared that this consciousness of self is a characteristic of human mentality; but, so far as self-consciousness in relation to the various parts of the body is concerned, it is possible to observe the development of this function in animals. The kitten does not realize for some time that its tail is part of itself, just as the infant is not aware of his relation to his own toe; yet the lesson is eventually learnt by both.

It is obvious that this development of awareness of self as an individual is an early event in the history of mankind, and one which has gone on developing through the ages. This resulted in a differentiation between the ego and the environment, and yet it was necessary to postulate some sort of connexion or intermediary. Thus arose the concept of the soul. Inevitably, at that stage of intellectual development when abstract thought was impossible, this concept was materialistic. If the self could recognize the hand as part of itself, then there must be two selves, independent of each other, and indistinguishable from each other, and so the differentiation arose between the self as knower and the self as known. This distinction gradually developed into an antagonism between soul and body, which was the basis of much religious controversy. What was this soul, this *alter ego*, was the question which occupied every one of the earlier thinkers. In early times it was envisaged as a shade, which interpenetrated the substance of the body, and which, when the body decayed, lived on in some other world. Professor Tylor[1] quotes a definition held by our ancestors as follows: "It is a thin unsubstantial human image, in its nature a sort of vapour, film or shadow, the cause of life and thought in the individual it animates; independently possessing the personal consciousness and volition of its corporeal owner, past or present; capable of leaving the body far behind, to flash swiftly from place to place; mostly impalpable and invisible, yet also manifesting physical power, and especially appearing to men, waking or asleep, as a phantasm, separate from the body, of which it bears the likeness, continuing to exist and appear to man after the death of that body, able to enter into, possess and act in the bodies of other men, of animals, and even of things." Such was the conception of those who could not think, except in terms of matter—matter which might be very tenuous and vague, but which had a definite substance as well as being.

And so the concept grew, fostered by the overwhelming impulse of self-expression and self-exaltation. The normal human being was naturally dissatisfied with the limitations and failures of this life, and demanded a better chance in another existence. So, he argued, it must be true that his soul lived on after him. A recent expression of this wish for immortality—the father of the thought—was that of a distinguished professor who considered that this belief was eminently satisfactory, because those who held it, could later meet the sceptics, and point out to them their errors; whereas, if survival was not true, there was no chance of a sceptic exulting over the credulous folly of the believer. Thus, the efforts of the later philosophers were mainly directed towards explaining the nature of the soul in such a way as to make its already accepted quality of immortality acceptable. This conception is modified in its turn by the envy, hatred, and malice felt towards the other members of the community. It was all very well for one's own soul to go on developing from height to height and to enjoy the fruits of Paradise, but surely such joys cannot be allowed to the man who robbed one's orchard or killed one's cow! Thus came the trials and punishments of after life. With the greater development of self-consciousness came the origin of the ego ideal, and with it, the realization that this was not reached. So there developed self-criticism which, under the influence of the early fear of the Gods, resulted in the application of future punishment to the self. Such ideas in relation to the soul were fostered by the teachings of the priests, who thereby achieved power over their neighbours and gain to themselves.

The concept of the vaguely material interpenetrating shade worked well, so long as the structure of the body was a matter of conjecture, but when anatomy became a relatively popular science, this did not fit in with the newly observed facts. From this a tendency arose to provide the soul with a more definite structure. Hence came the effort to find the site of the soul. Driven from pillar to post, from heart to liver, from liver to brain, the unfortunate homunculus found rest for a time in the pineal-gland, which was supposed to be the centre of the brain and the point to which all afferent impulses came, and from which all efferent impulses flowed. But even this last refuge was denied, and the only conclusion that could be entertained by the materialistic anatomist was, that the soul is non-existant, that immortality is a myth, and that there is nothing but the body. This body is composed of a collection of cells which eventually decompose, when, except for the energy liberated by the said decomposition, everything connected with the individual is lost to the universe. But in this analytic effort to find the soul, man was failing to see the wood for trees. As was so often the case, in this phase of the progress of knowledge man turned his whole attention to analysis and failed to understand the synthesis. In the effort to dispense with the soul, the strict materialist was depriving the majority of mankind of a necessity of life.

Naturally, the Church has always attempted to insist on the existence of a soul, as it is an essential feature of its teaching and its power. As usually expressed, however, even this conception is definitely materialistic, and the majority of people do not make much attempt to avoid Deification of the spiritual side of the personality, since all thinking tends to be in terms of objective things, except in the extreme introvert type. In the Middle Ages the concept was wholly materialistic, as witness the saying of St. Jerome: "If the dead be not raised with flesh and bones, how can the damned after judgment gnash their teeth in hell?" This is not to say that the Church is not perfectly justified in this teaching, for it must teach in the language that its disciples understand, but if thinking is to be really clarified, we must get rid of the material dress of true immaterial spiritualities.

With the existence of a soul, and its adventures after the death of the body, we have no direct concern, but this question of the philosophy of life and the immaterial aspect of personality is of some moment. If a spiritual relationship is sought, then it is clear that the physical aspects of our study need not concern us, and it is to the psychical aspect that we must direct our attention. It has been said that the study of personality is not complete unless the relationship of the whole with the environment has been taken into account, and it is in this relationship looked at from the psychical aspect, that the spiritual significance of the personality lies. A person's cognition and affection are largely individual matters, but the influence he exerts outside himself is brought about by conation. Moreover, the tendency in modern psychology is to regard conation as the significant part of mental processes. In considering this conation or behaviour, it must be realized that the personality finds touch with his environment, in virtue of his organization as a whole. To put it in another way, the individual reacts with his environment by his behaviour all through life. The various patterns of behaviour throughout the life of an individual are not a mere conglomeration, but emerge, as a definite unified entity. This emergence, like every other emergence, depends on, and involves its component parts. Moreover, all the factors which have been successively studied as components of personality, modify and are essential to the total organized pattern of behaviour.

Let us recapitulate. A man's behaviour certainly depends on, and is modified by the organization of his bodily function. Disease and injury alter the whole aspect of a man's relation to his environment. Inherent under-development or over-development of any given organ, or part of the body, makes a difference to his reactions. This is specially the case with the nervous system. The late war has shown us how utterly different men are, before and after a head wound ; indeed, if this is at all severe, the character is entirely changed, and can never resume its former nature. So behaviour is altered by the temperamental factor, especially in relation to the endocrine glands. The change in the individual who suffers from under or over function of the thyroid has been described already. Similarly, the cessation of function of the sex glands produce such marked modifications that it is referred to in popular speech as the change of life. The organization of mental function makes still more difference to this emergent. The proportion of his inherent dispositions, the organization or want of organization, into sentiments and beliefs, the value of these sentiments and beliefs, play the most important parts. Similarly, the question as to how the mind is orientated in relation to the sex impulses or in accordance with the ego impulse, or the creative impulse, determines the individual's behaviour. The general pattern of autonomic tensions has also been seen to have an influence. Again, in estimating this pattern of behaviour, we have to ask, Is the personality instable within itself, or towards the environment, is it dissociated or is it retarded? And only when we have considered all these factors in themselves and in their special relatedness to each other, can we understand and estimate this new emergent, the complex pattern of behaviour. This pattern further must be considered as a whole in virtue of its organization, which alone gives its significance. Indeed, as Holt[2] has pointed out, it is only in virtue of its organization as a whole, and considered as a going concern, that anything has a significance. A printing-press is a meaningless collection of rollers and wheels, of nuts and screws, unless these are organized in relation to their general function. So, individual patterns of behaviour, selected at random, are of no significance, but the whole emergent pattern of behaviour is of enormous significance, and once treated as a whole, it becomes evident that no one part can, or ought to be, considered by itself, since every part is interdependent and only has a significant meaning, when thought of in relation to the rest.

This emergent pattern of behaviour is what the individuality has achieved, and the impress made by him on the environment. This, which involves and depends on the whole material personality, is itself immaterial; it is a spiritual entity, but inseparable from a material entity, and is what may be described as the spiritual aspect of personality. This impress on the environment is the function of the personality, and gives the personality its significance in the general scheme of the universe. Without function, structure has little or no significance, once life has emerged. No doubt the structure of a crystal is its chief significance, but the structure of the heart, within the body, is of no significance compared with its function, yet the latter is of the most essential importance to the body.

It remains to consider what is the exact significance of this spiritual emergent. It is suggested that it has far more significance and importance than any other aspect of our subject. The materialistic bias of the last century has tended to confine the law of cause and effect to material influences, which can be appreciated by the senses. But it is quite clear that this view is too limited. The whole behaviour of a man has an enormous influence on his environment, not only in the present, but in the future. The universe is not a rigid structure, but a fluid process, if such a term be allowed, exquisitely sensitive to every influence, however small its amplitude. Thus, the emergent pattern of behaviour of any individual does mould the whole of existence. This influence, in the case of man, is made of infinitely greater significance than that of the animals, by his highly organized power of discriminative action, by the manipulative capacity of his hands, by the power of reflective thought, and above everything, by language. Without these, the influence he exerts is infinitesimal. Even the tiger can only influence his mate, his offspring and his prey, but the least of men has a radius of action immeasurably greater. The almost limitless possibilities of such influence may be grasped when we consider such men as Homer, Aristotle, Plato, Cæsar, Leonardo, Shakespeare, Goethe, Napoleon and, to descend to lesser lights, William Hohenzollern. This immaterial aspect of personality, which is not only the essential and fundamentally important emergent for the present, extends on into the future, continuing as an active, living influence, according to the greatness or littleness, the significance or insignificance of its organization. Nor is it possible, as has been said before, to detach units from this emergent entity. For example, it might be said, that we may take a play of Shakespeare, and admit that Hamlet survives and goes on exerting its influence down the ages; but without the whole personality of Shakespeare, Hamlet could not have been. Hamlet involved and depended on Shakespeare's bodily organization, his endocrine glands, his mental organization and the rest, and it is Shakespeare and not Hamlet that lives, that gives us pleasure and pain, modifies and rearranges our thoughts, and even may influence our daily actions.

Our next question must be, what relation has our spiritual personality, or our emergent pattern of behaviour, to our philosophy of life? In our study of the scheme on which personality is evolved we postulated an intervenient deity, as well as the quality of deity, to which end evolution proceeds. The quality of deity involves an emergent of the widest radius of activity which it is possible to conceive, so that the highest degree of harmony may exist in the universe. In this way we may expect that the lower selfish impulses, which limit man's altruistic behaviour, will all be sublimated on to the highest level of beauty, goodness and truth. Further, we may expect and hope, that this is the goal to which humanity is proceeding. By intervenient deity, we mean that this process of evolution is not going on in a purely haphazard way, without guidance or direction, but that all through the process, every component part is subject to a definite law, according to which evolution proceeds. Whether we are content to think of this law as an abstract conception, or whether we deify it, so that it becomes the command of a personal anthropomorphic God, or a more vague principle of nature, is of little importance, so long as we concede that humanity is progressing to a state of greater harmony, that is, of greater beauty, truth and goodness, and that it is proceeding thus according to definite laws, which we may strive to understand as best we may.

The philosophy of life of the majority is, therefore, that so far as possible, our emergent pattern of behaviour should be organized so that it accords with the law of intervenient deity and aims at emergence of the quality of deity. The question may at this point be raised, can we ourselves do anything to so organize our spiritual personality at all? This involves the vexed question of "freedom of will" which, as Locke said long ago "is not proper whether the will be free, but whether the man be free." For metaphysics, this may be of the greatest importance, but for psychology it is of much less moment. One point which generally confuses the issue must be ruled out at once. Freedom has no relation to responsibility. With the latter we are not concerned at all. Next, freedom, as Ward[1] has pointed out, may be external or internal. Man is essentially externally free, and indeed life itself, to a large extent, involves this external freedom. By this term is meant that the animal, by virtue of its organization, is no longer the sport of circumstances, as is the inanimate object, swept about by all that comes in contact with it, without power of response or choice. This choice is of course more objective than subjective. For instance, when a man takes a certain part, writes a book, or commits a crime, the observer says that he did this, though he might have done the opposite; yet the man's behaviour depends on the pattern of stimuli presented to him, on the organization of his mental and bodily function, and the resultant pattern of behaviour. When Martin Luther took his decision at the Diet of Worms, the observer and the historian think that he might have remained in the body of the church, and yet Luther himself said, "Ich kann nicht anders." Again, Luther might have recanted, like Galileo, but he didn't; he was not built that way. In virtue of his organization, then, man is externally free: is he in any way internally free? This is a more difficult question, and internal freedom involves a higher emergence, that of reflective thought. It is certain that those animals whose bodily organization knows no higher level than the thalamencephalon or basal ganglia and whose behaviour is consequently on the level of pure instinct have no internal freedom. They are bound by their organization to perfectly definite and determined lines of conduct. In man, however, there has evolved a cortex, and with the cortex the function of discrimination, reflective thought, and self-consciousness, all of which constitute what is known as conscience. As Ward says:

> "'It is true of Brutes that they
> Can like, but not distinguish too,
> Nor their own liking by reflection know.'

But it is not true of man as a rational being. Raised to the trans-subjective standpoint, through intercourse with his fellows, he has within his reach the gift to see himself as others see him. He has in consequence, a standard by which to estimate even himself; he can by taking thought, add to his mental, and still more to his moral stature; he may now have an ideal, and he can determine *proprio motu* to strive to realize it." It will be remembered, that even at the reflex level every pattern of behaviour served as a stimulus pattern which starts another cycle; and that, at the conscious level, this was so organized, that consciousness could never be truly regarded as static, but always as a process, each event in consciousness bending back to the past and leaning forward to the future, as successive engrams became activated. With the advent of the power of discrimination, of reflective thought, and self-consciousness, this law becomes of enormous importance, and every thought and every action is a stimulus pattern, which inevitably moulds and changes character. In virtue of this organisation lies man's internal freedom which "is not only negative but positive, not mere freedom from constraint, but freedom to initiate, to turn circumstances to account, even—thanks to the ποῦ στῶ that reason affords—so to deal with oneself." So, it is possible for man to mould the spiritual aspect of his personality in accordance with the philosophy of life he has adopted, and thereby gain that organization of sentiment and belief with relation to the universe, which alone permits the personality to be efficient, complete and content.

In virtue of this freedom, therefore, man has some power to mould and influence his emergent pattern of behaviour—his spiritual life, and therefore his responsibility to the future. It is in respect of this emergent pattern that he survives. It is in respect of this, that he helps or hinders God—the intervenient deity. It is in respect of this, that he approaches or recedes from the quality of deity—that he attains Godhead. It is this function of the synthesized complete personality that gives him significance. It is possible that here we may discover the secret of the soul, the secret of immortality, and the secret of communion with God. The answers to these riddles may be found, not in the realm of structure, but in that of function. May it be that the soul is not a part of the structure of the body, as the ancients believed, nor a function of that body, but the function of the total emergent personality which goes on exerting its influence through the ages, just in so far as its activities have altered the form of the universe. In some cases this influence is widespread, in others it is extremely local, but no one can live in the world without making some impression on the form of the universal whole.

REFERENCES

CHAPTER I

1. W. McDougall, *Social Psychology*. London, 1917.
2. J. Buchan, *The Path of the King*. London, 1920.
3. S. Laing, *Human Origins*. London, 1894.
4. Sir J. Frazer, *The Golden Bough*. London, 1923.
5. Sir C. Sherrington, *The Integrative Action of the Nervous System*. London, 1906.
6. Hughlings Jackson, *Papers on Aphasia* (reprinted). *Brain*, 1915, xxxviii.
7. H. Head, *Studies in Neurology*. London, 1920.
8. W. H. R. Rivers, *Instinct and the Unconscious*. Cambridge, 1920.
9. M. Wertheimer, "Experimentelle Studien über das Sehen von Bewegung," *Ztsch. f. Psychol.*, 1912, 61.
10. W. Köhler, *The Mentality of Apes* (International Library of Psychology). London & New York, 1925.
11. K. Koffka, "Perception : an Introduction to the Gestalt Theorie," *Psychol. Bull.*, 1922, xix, 10.
12. S. Alexander, *Space, Time and Deity*. 1920.
13. C. Lloyd Morgan, *Emergent Evolution*. London, 1923.
14. W. McDougall, *Body and Mind*. London, 1920.

CHAPTER II

1. W. McDougall, *Body and Mind*. London, 1920.
2. W. James, *Principles of Psychology*. London, 1920.
3. H. Bergson, *Matter and Memory*. London, 1920.
4. P. H. Huxley, *Essays*. London, 1893-4.
5. E. B. Holt, *The Concept of Consciousness*. London, 1914.
6. Bertrand Russell, *The Analysis of Mind*. London, 1921.
7. K. Koffka, "Introspection and the Method of Psychology" (*British Journal of Psychology*, 1924, xvi, 49).
8. R. Semon, *The Mneme*. London, 1916.
9. C. Lloyd Morgan, *Emergent Evolution*. London, 1923.
10. C. S. Myers, *Proceedings of the vii International Congress of Psychology at Oxford*, 1923.
11. Sir C. Sherrington, *Integrative Action of the Nervous System*. London, 1906.
12. Pawlow, *Atti del Congresso di Madrid*. 1904.
13. W. McDougall, *An Outline of Psychology*. London, 1923.

CHAPTER III

1. C. Lloyd Morgan, *Emergent Evolution*. London, 1923.
2. S. Alexander, *Space, Time and Deity*. London, 1920.
3. R. S. Lillie, *Protoplasmic Action and Nervous Action*. Chicago, 1923.
4. Reichart & Brown, *The Crystallography of Hæmoglobins*. Carnegie Institution Publications, No. 116, Washington, 1909.
5. G. H. Parker, *The Elementary Nervous System*. Philadelphia, 1918.
6. Sir C. Sherrington, *The Integrative Action of the Nervous System*. London, 1906.
7. W. H. R. Rivers, *Instinct and the Unconscious*. Cambridge, 1920,
8. C. Lloyd Morgan, *Instinct and Experience*. London, 1912.
9. W. McDougall, *An Outline of Psychology*. London, 1923.
10. R. Semon, *The Mneme*. London, 1916.

CHAPTER IV

1. Sir C. Sherrington, *Integrative Action of the Nervous System*. London, 1906.
2. R. Semon, *The Mneme*. London, 1916.
3. W. McDougall, *Social Psychology*. London, 1917.
4. H. Head, *Studies in Neurology*. Oxford, 1920.
5. S. A. Kinnier-Wilson, "Pathological Laughing and Crying" (*Jour. of Neurology and Psychopathology*, 1924, iv, 299).
6. L. Bianchi, *Mechanism of the Brain and the Function of the Frontal Lobes*. Edinburgh, 1922.

CHAPTER V

1. Leonard Williams, see *Proc. Royal Soc. of Med.*, 1923.
2. L. Guthrie and Emery, *Clinical Soc. Trans.*, 1907, xl, 175.
3. G. Pezard, see *Transactions of Brit. Assoc.* Liverpool, 1922.
4. F. E. Crew, *Trans. of Brit. Assoc.* Liverpool, 1923.
5. C. Herter, *Trans. Assoc. Amer. Phys.* 1908, xxiii, 260.
6. B. Bramwell, *Scot. Med. and Surg. Journal*, 1904, xiv, 321.
7. Hastings Gilford, *The Disorders of Postnatal Growth and Development*. 1911.
8. von Hansemann, *Berl. Klin. Wochensche.*, 1902, No. 52, p. 1209.
9. Sternberg, *Die Akromegalie und Vegetationsstörungen und Systemerkrankungen der Knochen* (Nothnagel, *Handb.*, vol. vii, Pt. II). Vienna, 1897-99.
10. Dieterle, *Jahrb. f. Kinderheilk.*, 1906, vol. 64, pp. 465 and 576.
11. A. Gigon, *Schweizer. Archiv. f. Neurol. und Psychol.*, ix, 2 (1921) and x, 1 (1922).
12. Stier, *Deutsche Zeitsch. f. Nervenheilk.*, 1912, vol. 44, p. 21.
13. Langdon Brown, *The Endocrine Glands* (*Brit. Med. Jl.* 1922, 1).
14. —— *The Sympathetic Nervous System in Disease*. London, 1924.

CHAPTER VI

1. W. McDougall, *An Outline of Psychology*. London, 1923.
2. L. Bianchi, *Mechanism of the Brain and the Function of the Frontal Lobes*. Edinburgh, 1922.
3. W. McDougall, *Social Psychology*. London, 1917.
4. J. Drever, *Instinct in Man*. Cambridge, 1917.
5. W. R. R. Rivers, *Instinct and the Unconscious*. Cambridge, 1920.
6. P. Janet, "La Tension Psychologique" (*Brit. Jl. of Psychol.:* Medical Sect., 1921).
7. J. Varendonck, *The Evolution of the Conscious Faculties*. London, 1923.

CHAPTER VII

1. P. Janet, "La Tension Psychologique" (*Brit. Jl. of Psychol.:* Medical Sect., 1921).
2. W. McDougall, *Social Psychology*. London, 1917.
3. A. F. Shand, *The Foundations of Character*. London, 1920.
4. J. Varendonck, *The Evolution of the Conscious Faculties*. London. 1923.
5. W. McDougall, *An Outline of Psychology*. London, 1923.

CHAPTER VIII

1. W. McDougall, *An Outline of Psychology*. London, 1923.
2. C. Jung, *Collected Papers on Analytical Psychology*. London, 1917,
3. W. Trotter, *Instincts of the Herd in Peace and War*. London, 1920.
4. W. McDougall, *National Welfare and National Decay*. London, 1921.
5. B. Hinkle, *The Re-creating of the Individual*. New York & London, 1924.
6. C. G. Seligman, *Anthropology and Psychology* (Presidential Address, Royal Anthropol. Inst., 1924).
7. Graham Wallas, *Our Social Heritage*. London, 1921.
8. J. Ward, *Psychological Principles*. Cambridge, 1920.

CHAPTER IX

1. S. Freud, *Traumdeutung*. Vienna, 1900.
—— *Drei Abhandlungen zur Sexualtheorie*. Vienna, 1905.
—— *Totem and Tabu*. London, 1919.
—— *Beyond the Pleasure Principle*. London, 1923.
—— *Group Psychology and the Analysis of the Ego*. London, 1923.
—— *Collected Papers*. London, 1925.

2. W. Trotter, *Instincts of the Herd in Peace and War*. London, 1920.
3. E. B. Holt, *The Freudian Wish*. London, 1917.
4. P. Janet, "La Tension Psychologique" (*Brit. Jour. of Psychol.: Med. Sect.*, 1921).
5. T. H. Pear, *Remembering and Forgetting*. London, 1922.
6. Sir J. Frazer, *The Golden Bough*. London, 1923.
7. D. Bryan, "The Freudian Psychology" (*Internat. Jl. of Psycho-anal.*, 1920).
8. H. Von Hug Helmuth, *A Study of the Mental Life of the Child*. Washington, 1919.

CHAPTER X

1. C. G. Jung, *Collected Papers on Analytical Psychology*. London, 1917.
   —— *Psychology of the Unconscious*. New York & London, 1916.
   —— *Psychological Types* (International Library of Psychology). London & New York, 1923.
2. R. Semon, *The Mneme*. London, 1916.
3. W. H. R. Rivers, *Instinct and the Unconscious*. Cambridge, 1920.
4. J. H. Van der Hoop, *Character and the Unconscious* (Intern. Lib. of Psychology). London & New York, 1923.
5. B. M. Hinkle, *The Recreating of the Individual*. New York & London, 1924.

CHAPTER XI

1. A. Adler, *The Neurotic Constitution*. London, 1904.
   —— *Study of Organ Inferiority and its Psychical Compensation*. New York, 1917.
   —— *Individual Psychology* (International Library of Psychology). London & New York, 1924.
2. C. Lloyd Morgan, *Emergent Evolution*. London, 1923.
3. Sir F. Mott, "Reproductive Organs in Relation to Mental Disorders" (*Brit. Med. Journal*, 1922, 1).
4. F. E. Crew, *Trans. of Brit. Assoc.* Liverpool, 1923.
5. E. C. Tolman, *Proc. of vii Internat. Congress of Psychol.* Oxford, 1923.
6. B. Hinkle, *The Recreating of the Individual*. New York & London, 1924.
7. H. Maeder, quoted in (6), p. 346.
8. I. Bloch, *The Sexual Life of our Time*. London, 1909.
9. Havelock Ellis, *Men and Women*. London, 1904.
10. S. Brierley. See *Internation. Journal of Psycho-analysis*, 1921.

CHAPTER XII

1. E. J. KEMPF, *The Autonomic Functions and the Personality* (Nerv. and Ment. Diseases Monograph Ser., No. 28).
—— *Psychopathology*. London, 1921.
2. Sir C. SHERRINGTON, in *Brain*, xxxviii, 1915, 191.
3. G. H. PARKER, *The Elementary Nervous System*. Philadelphia, 1918.
4. W. H. McDOUGALL, *An Outline of Psychology*. 1923.
5. Mosso. See GODDARD, *Psychology of the Normal and Subnormal*. New York & London, 1919.
6. W. CANNON, *Bodily Changes in Pain, Hunger, Fear, and Rage*. London, 1915.
7. Sir C. SHERRINGTON. See J. R. ANGELL, *Psychological Rev.*, 1916.

CHAPTER XIII

1. W. McDOUGALL, "The Revival of Emotional Memories and its Therapeutic Value" (*Brit. Jl. of Psychol.*: Med. Sect., 1, 1920).
2. W. H. R. RIVERS, *Instinct and the Unconscious*. Cambridge, 1920.
3. J. DREVER, *Instinct in Man*. Cambridge, 1917.
4. P. JANET, *The Major Symptoms of Hysteria*. New York, 1907.
5. L. BIANCHI, *Mechanism of the Brain and the Function of the Frontal Lobes*. Edinburgh. 1922.
6. W. TROTTER, *The Instincts of the Herd in Peace and War*. London, 1920.
7. W. JAMES, *Varieties of Religious Experience*. New York, 1899.
8. A. MAEDER, *Cure and Development in Psychic Life*. Zurich, 1915.
9. O. PFISTER, *Some Applications of Psycho-Analysis*. London, 1923.
10. G. GELEY, *De l'inconscient au conscient*. Paris, 1919.
11. G. DWELSHAUVERS, *L'Inconscient*. Paris, 1919.

CHAPTER XIV

1. C. LOMBROSO, *The Female Offender*.
2. C. GORING, *The English Convict* (Abridged Edit.). London, 1919.
3. W. HEALY, *Mental Conflicts and Misconduct*. New York & London, 1919.
—— *The Individual Delinquent*. New York & London, 1915.
4. C. BURT, "The Causes and Treatment of Juvenile Delinquency" (*Psyche*, 1922, 11, 232).
5. F. SHRUBSHALL, "The After History of Some Cases of Epidemic Encephalitis" (*Jour. of Neur. & Psychopath.*, iv, 236).
6. W. McDOUGALL, *Social Psychology*. London, 1917.
7. A. F. SHAND, *The Foundations of Character*. London, 1920.

CHAPTER XV

1. W. McDougall, *An Outline of Psychology*. London, 1923.
2. Morton Prince, *The Unconscious: the Fundamentals of Human Personality*. Boston, 1913.
3. C. G. Jung, *Collected Papers on Analytical Psychology*. London, 1917.
4. S. Freud, *Traumdeutung*. Vienna, 1900.
5. P. Janet, *The Major Symptoms of Hysteria*. New York, 1907.
6. Morton Prince, *The Dissociation of a Personality*. New York, 1906.
7. *Problems of Personality* (International Library of Psychology). London & New York, 1925.
8. S. Alexander, *Space, Time, and Deity*. 1920.

CHAPTER XVI

1. A. F. Tredgold, *Mental Deficiency*. London, 1914.
2. C. Spearman, *Amer. Journal of Psychology*, xv, 1904, 75.
3. A. Binet and Th. Simon, *A Method of Measuring the Development of Intelligence in Young Children*. Chicago, 1915.
4. L. M. Terman, *The Measurement of Intelligence*. London, 1919.
5. J. Varendonck, *The Evolution of the Conscious Faculties*. London 1923.
6. W. Kohler, *The Mentality of Apes* (International Library of Psychology). London & New York, 1924.
7. W. McDougall, *Social Psychology*. London, 1917.
8. W. James, *Text-Book of Psychology*. London, 1904.

CHAPTER XVII

1. E. B. Tylor, *Primitive Culture*, vol. 1, p. 420. London, 1871.
2. E. B. Holt, *The Freudian Wish*. London, 1917.
3. J. Ward, *Psychological Principles*. Cambridge, 1918.

INDEX

For Product Safety Concerns and Information please contact our EU representative GPSR@taylorandfrancis.com
Taylor & Francis Verlag GmbH, Kaufingerstraße 24, 80331 München, Germany

www.ingramcontent.com/pod-product-compliance
Lightning Source LLC
LaVergne TN
LVHW011115300926
849160LV00008B/387
* 9 7 8 1 1 3 8 8 7 5 3 8 8 *